The Autoimmune Warrior's Healing Key

Unlock your x-factor. Reclaim your life.

Jo Pronger Faulkner, BCom

Boondocks Publishing

Print ISBN: 978-1-7775628-0-9
1st Edition

TABLE OF CONTENTS

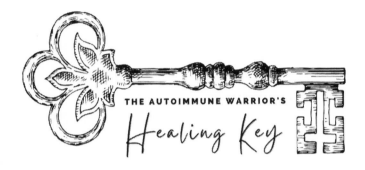

THE AUTOIMMUNE WARRIOR'S

Healing Key

ACKNOWLEDGMENTS

Have you ever read a book that thanked YOU? Yes, you! Whether we know each other or not, I want to take this opportunity to sincerely thank you for coming on this journey we are about to embark on together. When I was writing every single word, every single page, I felt you right along with me. I wrote this for you. I hope as you are reading, you feel like I'm right along with you, guiding you, encouraging you, giving you a kick in the pants once in a while, and celebrating your wins along the way.

Thank you to my *now fiancé* Mike: my best friend, my number one fan, my rock. A fun fact about us, for those of you who might not know, is that our parents were in each other's wedding parties, before either of us was born. When a friend you've known for your whole life becomes your life partner, it's pretty easy to believe it was meant to be. All the trials and tribulations that led me back to you were worth it. I'm so grateful to have a life as lucky as mine, with you alongside me for this amazing ride, and I love that you are as excited as I am about whatever is next.

I would also like to also thank my mum Lois Shand, Mike's mum Marlene Boone, Michele Imrie, Jennifer Winter, Lianne Waters, Erin Hollon, and editor C.B. Moore for your helpful feedback during the various drafts, and Lauren da Silva for your insights and thought-provoking questions. Each of your perspectives and suggestions guided me to write, re-write, and re-write again, making this book into the best version it could possibly be.

When considering who to ask to write the foreword for this book, Carol Howden was a clear choice. Not only is she a genuine, caring leader in natural wellness, she empowers everyone around her to believe in themselves and to take personal responsibility in all areas of their life. Thank you, Carol, for setting the bar high; for living life with curiosity, positivity, and intention, and inspiring me to do the same.

Thank you to my step-sister Samantha Hawkins for making my cover image look fabulous with your magic photo edits.

And last but not least, I would like to acknowledge my former rheumatologist, the late Dr. Jerry Tenenbaum. He came across as gruff sometimes but always appreciated my preparedness and questions. His busy practice, with back-to-back appointments all day, every day, was based solely on seeing patients who were very ill. Whenever I sat in his clinic waiting room, overhearing the many heart-breaking patient complaints, I imagined it probably wasn't a fun job. My gratitude towards him began in our first meeting when he took my illness very seriously, and got me on a treatment plan.

I appreciated him even more when, years later, he listened genuinely to my concerns about all the prescriptions I was taking. When I explained to him I wanted to try a different approach to my health, unlike others I told, he didn't shake his head and tell me it was impossible. He encouraged me to try it, and advised me to seek the assistance of my pharmacist for guidance in slowly weaning off my medications little by little, safely. I sure wish he could be here to see me now, to read this, and to know that I am grateful.

PREFACE

This book came to fruition after two years of answering questions from other women struggling with autoimmune conditions. We call ourselves "warriors" because we have been bravely fighting for a long time against a threat we can't even see.

I get asked in person. I get messages from total strangers. I get emails, phone calls and messages from friends and family saying their friend or colleague wants to hear my story.

What started as individual conversations turned into a blog post that got longer and longer. Then I wrote parts two and three of the blog post. I also created a multi-page, downloadable guide on my website, and later created a course, until finally I realized my experiences could become a very helpful book and it needed to be brought to life.

The more I was asked, "How did you do it?" the more I realized there are a great number of women looking for answers to their illness and to their desire for wellness, who don't seem to be able to find this information all in one place. And in North America, the over-arching advice comes from Western-trained medical professionals who want to treat the immediate issue at hand rather than investigate its cause or consider all the interconnected systems and overlapping symptoms.

I truly hope you don't have to experience the lows that I did. They were nearly the death of me. I was really sick for a long time, and frustrated by a lack of answers from so many people whose help I sought. My autoimmune symptoms were dismissed by the first few doctors I saw; I was laughed at when describing some of my symptoms I was worried about; I was disbelieved, told it was all in my head; and when I finally got what I thought were answers, I was told the disease was a lifelong diagnosis that not many people knew much about.

After my fourth autoimmune diagnosis, topped off with skin cancer, I felt a strong conviction that there must be an underlying reason for what my body was doing. The idea that each health issue was independent of the others didn't sit well with my analytical mind.

I needed some different answers, and so I went looking for them myself.

I hope learning about my journey and what I ultimately discovered can help you in your journey too.

~ Jo Pronger Faulkner

FOREWORD

There is nothing that touches one's heart like hearing the story of someone's personal journey of overcoming all odds. To truly understand the root cause, that the body is the manifestation of the mind, and then move into action, Jo Pronger Faulkner is truly an inspiration.

Most of us grow up with the idea that if you eat right and exercise, you will be healthy. As we get older, we can get caught up in the idea that following the latest diet, or working out for an hour a day is what we need to do to get or to stay healthy. The problem with these approaches is twofold: firstly, there is no one-size-fits-all solution to health. Each person has different tolerances and needs. Secondly, and more importantly, neither approach addresses the root cause of what our health challenges are.

Jo Pronger Faulkner introduces you to principles and ideas about health that aren't anything like the ones you grew up with. However, marvelous things can begin to happen as you start to incorporate these new ideas into your life, even if you have experienced symptoms of ill health for years. With the right formula, a body that's in a state of "dis-ease" can be transformed into a body "at-ease."

In the short time I have interacted with Jo, I have such admiration for her passion and dedication to helping people live healthy, happy and prosperous lives. I'm very proud to know and work with her.

5

I was very pleased when she told me that she had written a book, because I know she has helped many of her friends and family succeed in their lives. And now, through this book she can expand her reach to help even more people transform their health, and their entire outlook on life.

I personally have studied the principle of success for over two decades. This study helped me to realize in order to be successful in any area of your life, from being healthy to achieving wealth, loving relationships, and a fulfilling career, you must work in harmony with Universal Laws that control the results you get in life.

Jo has woven the essence of those principles into her life and into this book. She provides a system for implementing any change you'd like to make in your life, along with the basic tools and principles for how to create a healthy body. When you follow the system, you won't just get temporary improvements; you will get lasting results.

I clearly remember when I was introduced to the fact that, "we become what we think about", this phrase shifted my perspective and put me on a journey that changed my life forever. I still study these *principles and laws of the universe* every single day. The ideas in this book reflect the same principles and will help you on your journey of wellness.

Unlike many books about health and success, Jo does not suggest eating a rigid and restrictive diet, and exercising for a set number of minutes every day as a way to enjoy a healthier life. Instead, she provides a system of getting to the root of your physical and mental symptoms and creating the right path for you, the one that can lead you to health, joy, and abundance in every area of your life.

However, as powerful as the ideas in this book are, simply reading each page will not improve your health, or change anything in your life. You must act on the ideas to get the results that you want. Jo has outlined action steps for you to take at the end of each chapter. I suggest you do exactly this, and get ready for an exciting journey and a healthy new you.

~ Carol Howden, *Young Living Royal Crown Diamond, Proctor Gallagher Consultant, Author of Ancient Wisdom in Modern Menu*

CHAPTER ONE

My Story

In October 2010, I got sick. At first it was H1N1 — the "swine flu." It was the worst flu I've ever had, knock on wood. I was really down and out, with all the classic symptoms, and I was off work for nearly two weeks. Quite a few people in my community also had it, including one friend who ended up in the hospital for a day or two. After a few weeks I seemed to get better, for the most part. I was able to go back to work, at least, but when I tried to resume my fitness classes I was still too drained to really participate. For months afterwards, I felt like I hadn't fully recovered and still had a touch of the flu.

I ran out of breath more quickly than I knew I should. My shoulders ached deep down inside, and nothing I did or took for pain relief helped. In January 2011, I went on a tropical vacation to Jamaica because I knew a week in the hot weather would solve all my problems. Except, it didn't.

As I lay on the beach in a comfy lounge chair that felt like it was made just for me, listening to the gentle ocean waves lapping against the hot sand and drinking my umpteenth piña colada, I remember thinking, *"Why do my shoulders still hurt? I shouldn't be feeling anything at this point!"*

It was the very moment when I came to a dreadful realization something wasn't right. I got that butterfly feeling in the pit of my stomach. My vacation suddenly got stressful. The thought just wouldn't leave my mind. I knew something was wrong.

I was held up returning the rental car at the airport, and the plane began boarding without me. My adrenaline was in high gear as I ran through a large section of the Montego Bay International Airport, with my backpack full of clothes, flip flops, souvenirs and carefully padded little bottles of rum flopping around on my back. I became so short of breath and my lungs hurt so much as I gasped to breathe that I had to stop. I literally bent over in the middle of the airport hallway, vacant by that point because everyone heading towards that boarding gate was on the plane. I couldn't seem to get enough air and decided it was totally fine that I was missing my plane since I was about to have a couple of exploded lungs anyway. I still remember the pain to just breathe.

It wasn't like I was out of shape. Despite previously suffering from effects of complex regional pain syndrome starting in 2007 when I broke my leg in four places, I had been gradually improving my fitness. I completed a full year of physiotherapy, massage treatments, and from the time I was off crutches after my surgery, I also regularly saw a chiropractor for adjustments. All of these therapies were beneficial in my healing, posture, and strength-building. In early 2008, I was "graduated" by my physiotherapist — told I didn't need any further treatments — when the leg I had broken became stronger than my other one!

Fast forward a couple of years: for much of 2010, up until my H1N1 episode, I had been going to boxing classes twice a week; in the summer I added a cardio exercise class once a week, and was doing five-mile trail runs at least once a week, sometimes twice. I had even been able to do seventy-five push-ups (real ones!) in a friendly competition against my stepson. I actually felt like I was in the best physical shape ever, other than this new sensation like I was about to die.

I did manage to catch my flight out of Jamaica. And after I got home, my thyroid basically quit. By the end of January 2011, I became so lethargic and groggy at times, sometimes I forgot words and just stopped talking mid-sentence. I felt like my brain and my body were shutting down at the same time. A doctor at my local walk-in clinic told me I was depressed and needed talk therapy. He put me on an antidepressant. My intuition on this was strong, though — I knew that wasn't the issue. I just didn't yet know what it was.

I kept going to other doctors and pushing for tests. After a few months a new doctor discovered my thyroid was low (known as hypothyroidism), so he put me on a synthetic hormone regulator for the thyroid gland. I'm sure he thought he had solved my problem.

"You'll be fine, just keep coming in every three months for a blood test and prescription renewal." He told me more than once I would be on these pills forever. I was only thirty-eight years old.

"Forever? Really?" It seemed so final.

But it wasn't just my thyroid, so the levothyroxine pills didn't solve everything. I came back to my doctor every couple of weeks with lists of additional complaints: headaches, blotchy red rashes over my entire torso (front and back), rashes on the insides of my arms, up the sides of my breasts, across my upper chest, across the front and sides of my neck, and sometimes up the sides of my face to my forehead. None of the rash episodes were itchy, but they carried some heat to them, and they were alarming to look at. I also had deep internal joint pain, no energy, bladder pressure and twinges, extremely painful menstrual periods, and randomly-occurring, stabbing eye pain. I would lose my voice for days at a time like I had laryngitis, and other miscellaneous, strange issues. I caught every cough or cold my co-workers or friends had. These coughs turned into seal-barking, phlegm-hacking bronchitis for me, almost every time.

I began to get embarrassed about all of my symptoms because there were so many; they would come and go, and they seemed unrelated. I was pretty sure I was dying from some mysterious rare disease. My doctor was running a busy walk-in medical practice and told me one day he could only address one complaint at a time (per appointment). I started to worry that he thought I was a hypochondriac and wouldn't believe that I was sick. So I started to pick and choose what I would bring up at my appointments — usually it was a toss-up between what made me feel the worst, or what I was feeling at the time of my appointment. And with only being able to talk about one symptom, if it was a headache or PMS, guess how quickly those got brushed off! On multiple occasions when I asked about my rashes (I even brought a photograph of my latest one with me one day), he would always say it was most likely an allergy to my laundry soap. When I said I had no energy, he said, "Try getting more sleep," and then gave me a prescription for sleeping pills.

Little did the doctors know, and little did I know,
my body was in a full-blown systemic malfunction.

Meanwhile, I was also experiencing long-term, chronic stress from multiple angles. My marital relationship was a roller coaster. Several years earlier, I had decided to go to university for a bachelor's degree, and my partner's negative reaction to me wanting to better myself should have been a red flag. From then on, we bounced back and forth from pretending everything was storybook magical to being on a verge of a break-up — while trying to hide my packed boxes of belongings from the kids and extended-family members with whom we shared the house. These cycles usually occurred every six to eight months and went on for years. When I wanted to leave, I was guilted into staying. Then, when I decided to stay and wasn't happy, he would remind me that I was the one who "chose to stay." Everything seemed to be my fault no matter what.

The longer we were together, the more intertwined our personal and financial lives became, and the harder it got to make the looming decision. We had a house on a little acreage because since I was ten years old I dreamed of having my own horse, and I had also hoped a horse would help bring me and my stepdaughter closer together. For much of my adulthood I've also had a financial goal to have rental properties for future (retirement) security, and by the time I got really sick, we owned four properties together. Life gets messy.

Meanwhile with workplace drama and a 90-minute commute each way to the city and back, I felt like a piece of me was dying inside every day. I felt stuck and powerless. I felt like I was outside my life looking in, heading for burnout and couldn't figure out how to stop it.

I'm a numbers girl, and I enjoyed the budget management and financial analysis I was doing, but unfortunately I worked closely with several people who were negative, manipulative, condescending, and would be the first to throw their staff and colleagues under the bus if anything went sideways. One of the managers — a very feisty woman who was outspoken, and an obvious red personality type — would run in our cubicle hallways to go back and forth between other managers' offices. Whenever she was standing still (usually just long enough to yell at my boss through his open door twenty feet from my cubicle), she would unknowingly flap her arms. Humor has always been one of my coping mechanisms, and I tried to draw her attention to her behavior in a non-confrontational way by making jokes like, "No running in the halls!" but she would just glare at me.

It was a chaotic work environment. You could cut the tension with a knife most days. Several people in our division took early retirement, and sick leave among the remaining staff was common. Most of my colleagues regularly applied on as many job postings as they could find in other branches until they could get out, and due to organizational shuffling I ended up with the arm-flapper as my boss. Her energy was intense.

My insides were in constant fight-or-flight mode, at home and at work. I got sicker and sicker, with no answers in sight. Many people at the office, other than a couple of close friends, thought I was faking an illness just to get out of coming to work. What they didn't see was that on the days I did not go to work, I couldn't get out of bed before noon, I often had trouble keeping food down, a pounding headache, eye pain and blurred vision that would come and go, I felt dizzy and disoriented (making driving and thinking difficult), had random body and joint pain, and began to have trouble concentrating, especially on details (reading spreadsheets and emails were challenging).

14

My thoughts became scattered. My ability to think critically was fogged over. I sometimes wondered if I had Alzheimer's disease or dementia. Or mercury poisoning. Or a parasite infestation. When you don't know where to begin, and have no idea what could possibly be wrong, it's a dark, lonely place.

It took eighteen months of weekly doctor appointments, specialist appointments relating to specific symptoms, and many months of missed work to finally get referred to a rheumatologist. By then I had seen an ear-nose-throat specialist for my voice hoarseness which, via a small telescope, revealed inflamed vocal cords; a urologist for my bladder issues which, with an ultrasound, showed a uterine fibroid that caused me pain and excess bleeding; and an MRI for my low back pain which revealed a bulged disc. I had also seen many other doctors and specialists whose various test and examination results were decidedly "normal."

The rheumatologist diagnosed me immediately as having lupus when he looked at the stack of about twenty rash photographs I had brought to the appointment the first time I saw him, and after listening to me read a handwritten list of all the symptoms I had been dealing with.

He followed up his expert opinion with an in-depth blood panel specifically looking for autoimmune antibodies. My ANA (antinuclear antibody) test came back positive, which when combined with all my other symptoms meant I was dealing with systemic lupus erythematosus. Believe it or not, I felt relieved! Who says this about an autoimmune diagnosis?

My wave of relief came from finally feeling validated and confirmed — I wasn't making it up, I was actually really sick and had a real disease name. Now a diagnosis could be proven through formal medical documentation for my supervisor, friends and even some family members who doubted me. I would be able to have my disability claim approved and get back pay for many months of missed work with zero income.

I was put on Plaquenil (hydroxychloroquine), which is a typical immune-suppressing drug used for lupus. This just added to the handful of pills I was already taking for complex regional pain syndrome, depression, and hypothyroidism. I also randomly took sleeping pills every few nights (I was worried about becoming addicted, but on nights I didn't take them I didn't sleep). I frequently needed antibiotics for recurring urinary tract and lung infections, as well as daily over-the-counter pain relief medications.

In all my appointments with medical professionals, before my diagnosis and after, not one of them ever said anything about nutrition, or about trying to get to the root cause of why I was sick. None of them ever seemed concerned about the growing number of pills I was taking at my relatively young age. It seemed every time I saw a new doctor, I came out of the clinic with an additional prescription, having been shoved one rung down on the ladder of hope.

I cried a lot. *"How could this really be my life?"*

In 2014, a few months after the very stressful final break up from the volatile marital relationship I'd been in, I also began to test positive on the extractable nuclear antibody (ENA) test: I now had mixed connective tissue disease on top of everything else.

FOUR autoimmune diseases by age forty-one.

I was newly single, struggling financially, hanging onto my stressful career by a thread, in the beginning of what was becoming an ugly legal battle because my ex wanted to keep all our shared properties for himself, and I was devastated.

I will never forget the day I got a follow-up phone call from my general practitioner to give me the news about now having MCTD. He sounded scared for me. I was his first patient with lupus, and he already had a hard enough time trying to figure out what to do with me. Now here was another autoimmune disease neither of us knew anything about.

I was sure it was a death sentence. One more nail in my half-built coffin. I quietly ended the call, held the phone to my chest, and numbly stared out my living room window at my beautiful horse in his paddock — the love of my life. Not even bothering to wipe away my tears, I wondered what would happen to him when I died.

CHAPTER TWO

Decisions and Outcomes

There's a scene in the 1998 movie *Meet Joe Black* that brings tears to my eyes every time I watch it. The birthday scene on its own won't mean much if you haven't seen the entire movie, and honestly the first time I watched it I thought it was weird. Yet the concept behind the story began to marinate in my head. The next time I watched it, I surprised myself when my eyes welled up and I got a lump in my throat.

I've seen this movie now countless times, and the birthday scene breaks me up inside. Every damn time.

In front of a huge crowd of friends and family,
the dad, William Parrish (played by Anthony Hopkins),
blows out the solo candle on the top of
his oversized birthday cake.

He takes a moment to compose himself,
and says matter-of-factly that he is going to confess
his one-candle wish. He tells his party guests his desire is
that they could have a life as lucky as his; that he hopes they
reach "the end" feeling blessed and satisfied, knowing
they did not want anything else out of life.

We all want to live our best lives, don't we? I want to have lived it all, lived it by my own design and by my own choosing. Not in a material way, but experientially, and with meaning. With people riding along whom I chose to let in on the fun.

The irony is we don't stumble across a lucky life by chance. People who appear to be lucky have created it for themselves through:

Learning about beliefs, forgiveness, and mindset;
Understanding themselves and others on a deep level;
Curiosity about everything, whether they like it, agree with it, or not; and
Knowledge gained by summoning their courage to experience new things.

Life is precious, and it really is shorter than we think. Autoimmune illness tries to steal it from us.

Six years after my last autoimmune diagnosis, I no longer call them diseases. To me, they were malfunctions. Yes, past tense. I have reversed them, turned my health right-side up, and am sharing everything I did with you so you can too.

One of the most significant epiphanies I had after experiencing relief from most of my symptoms is that *this is a lifestyle*. And what made me realize this was whenever I would slide back into old habits just a little, I would begin to feel symptoms again within a short period of time.

My body will malfunction again if I revert to my old ways, but why would I — why would anyone — want to? We don't know what we don't know, but once we know better, we can DO better if we have the right tools and know what they are used for.

Getting better starts with *being* better. And that means becoming unstuck from our emotional programming and committing to a plan. For us autoimmune warriors, these aren't topics to take lightly. It feels harder than you want it to be. Especially when you're already exhausted. I get it.

The biggest hurdle to overcome is your own limiting beliefs. If you are feeling powerless, this is simply a false reality of yours that is holding you back. Do you believe you are worthy of living the life you once dreamed of? Self-worth is a really challenging self-reflection exercise for a lot of women. Do you believe you just "get what you get," and need to "play the cards you were dealt," or do you believe that you can change the rules of the game so that everyone wins?

You can make a huge impact on your own life. You are so much more than you have been taught to believe. I bet you have had some symptoms, or some ideas about improving your health, that you have been told aren't possible, or that have been brushed off by other people. One of the most important life lessons to learn is to trust your intuition. Start paying attention. Be curious about what your body feels like and what it is doing. Get quiet and really become aware. You'll know when something doesn't feel right — whether it's with your body, your health, your relationships, and everything else in life.

Friend, we each know more than we give ourselves credit for. It's just that we are often talked out of listening to our own intuition.

Your decisions, good and bad, have gotten you to where you are (no judgement here; I was in the same boat, remember?). I used to avoid listening to my intuition because of a saying I once heard about needing to think with your head, not your heart. It's rather a cold phrase and doesn't leave much room for feelings or compassion, does it? Limiting beliefs are often driving our decision-making processes, and can really make a mess of things!

Every "next" choice you make, day after day, can get you closer to where you want to go if you set a goal and start focusing on it. Or it can take you further from it. You have the power every minute of every day to change your outcome and write your own story from this point forward.

I'm not going to sugarcoat this. It's not easy, but it's so worth it.

It really doesn't matter which malfunction you are having — there are common denominators to the perfect storm of what contributes to autoimmune illness. I didn't do specific, different things for each of my four diagnoses. I did all the things you are going to learn about, and my malfunctioning endocrine system began to normalize again.

Recently, a friend asked me the source of my "radical discipline" superpower. I got goosebumps. I've been told many times that I'm too headstrong, too stubborn, too hardcore or too focused. Too "something," in a judgmental tone.

For decades, well into adulthood, I've tried to shine less brightly around certain people because my past shining moments of drive and determination were met with insults or condescending remarks that stung at the time, and for years afterward. They played in a loop in my head, validating my own insecurities and limiting beliefs. This emotional turmoil only added to my chronic stress.

My guess is you've been teased or shamed about whatever your special superpower or lane of genius is too. Friend, embrace the things that make you YOU. You are worthy, you are deserving, and you have unique gifts to share!

To consider that being radically disciplined is not common, and is not something everyone knows how to do, gave me pause. Could it be that people don't know how to be disciplined even when they want to be? This gave me renewed focus on how to help people not only with autoimmune illness, but every aspect of their lives.

I thought this might even be the x-factor
in my own healing journey and why
I've been able to get better while others who
also want to get better still struggle.

But this was only part of it.
I'm not radically disciplined about
everything. But I AM radically disciplined
about things that matter to me.

Have you been wanting to improve your health but not decided on a plan of action? You don't know what to change, and it's easier to stay in old habits, right? People do this in their finances, too, and in so many other aspects of their lives. A year may go by. Or five. They still say they want to improve this, that or the other and yet... they haven't. And when it comes to health or finances, trying to ignore the problem doesn't stop it from getting worse.

There comes a point in time when you can't keep delaying decisions. You're missing out on everything by not doing anything. Sometimes what feels easy, like eating the familiar food we know isn't good for us, or sitting on the couch scrolling social media for several hours a day, is just a distraction from doing hard, uncomfortable things. Our subconscious minds are hardwired to choose what feels "safe," familiar, and to take paths of least resistance (usually the most ingrained habits) because these are survival mechanisms.

It won't be easy. When it comes to changing the level of our wellness and getting better from a health — or even a financial — crisis, there isn't such thing as instant gratification. I think everyone realizes this deep down, yet still we secretly look for miraculous "quick fixes" we hope will change everything, or we get stuck not taking any steps at all.

I also desperately wanted to believe that once I knew what was causing my life to derail, I would get my health, my finances, and my life back on track immediately. I thought I wanted to know what was wrong with my health because once it had a label (a disease name) perhaps there would be a magic pill — a cure to make it all go away. It's devastating to watch your life crumble when you can't function very well anymore.

It's not autoimmune disease that is so debilitating;
it's the symptoms and effects.

Be careful not to fool yourself into thinking there's an overnight fix for any health condition. Reality check: it took how many years to get to this point? You simply can't expect to feel back to your normal, pre-illness self after reading a few chapters in a book, thinking some positive thoughts, doing a yoga session and having a salad tonight for dinner.

This is a lifestyle, not a task that gets checked off your to-do list.

Not only is one autoimmune condition difficult to live with, but without making changes, chances are quite high you will add more overlapping disease symptoms as the years go by. Between 2007 and 2014, I was diagnosed with four specifically named autoimmune conditions. And then melanoma in late 2016.

I remember saying to my mother while awaiting biopsy results from the mole I had removed, "I've already got lupus, that's bad enough. What are the chances? Don't worry, I won't get cancer, too." I felt like I had enough on my plate and that the universe wouldn't hand me another health crisis. I mean, how many times could a person be kicked while they were down? Until I was told by my doctor that the results came back and I needed surgery immediately because they didn't get it all.

Are you wondering how someone could be so unlucky?

I will take you on my journey and show you how I figured out how to have less pain, less brain fog, better sleep, more energy, and relief from the daily struggles of autoimmune illness.

If you can learn what your symptoms are caused by, it'll give you a light at the end of the tunnel because you'll also learn how to avoid triggering many of those symptoms.

In turn I was able to improve my finances because I managed my expenses more purposefully, I was able to start working again, I made decisions on a couple of business ideas I had, and I was able to make some financial choices that hadn't even been a consideration when I was in the depths of my illness.

My friendships with a few special people who had stuck by me through chronic illness and highly stressful divorce were reinvigorated because I was reinvigorated. I have been able to experience a new love relationship where I am valued and respected for who I am, not who he wants me to be. And when I desired to change myself, better myself, learn new things, and even become an author, he supported me one hundred percent and has been my most enthusiastic cheerleader. Having the right people in your corner is truly priceless, and it's up to each of us to intentionally choose who to keep and who to distance ourselves from.

Through learning how to get my life back, I regained my confidence, set some boundaries, became the master of my own mojo and was finally able to embrace living a high-vibing, dream-building life.

This is what could be waiting for you above the wellness line too.

Turning your health right-side up again will take some really hard work, some painful (and hopefully also some joyful) self-discovery, and, yes, you may even shed some toxic tears of realization. I did. Just make sure you follow them up with forgiving yourself, and then promise to do your best for your body and mind from this point forward.

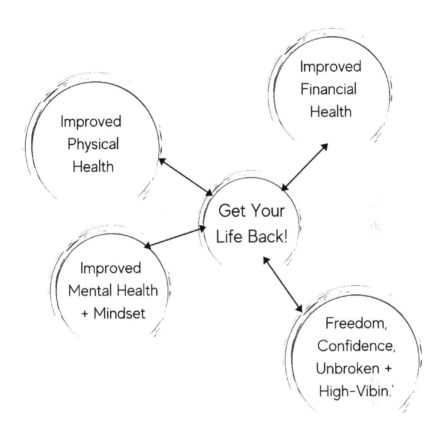

You may be thinking, "I don't know if I'm up for this."
For starters, you don't even know yet what "this" is.

And secondly, ask yourself, "What are the
consequences of waiting and doing nothing?"

Your physical health is on the line, your finances are in a downward spiral, and your relationships are suffering. How do I know? Because I've been there.

I've been where you are, and I know how seriously shitty it is to miss friends' Friday-night social gatherings, or kids' hockey-tournament games, or to miss multiple days (or weeks or months) of work.

I know what it's like to have no motivation, no vitality, no happiness, to just want to get it over with and die already, and to have no hope. I thought about ending my life quite a few times. I weighed the pros and cons of that decision too, and tried to figure out a way that would be minimally chaotic and traumatizing for whoever found me. I couldn't come up with a solid plan on how to do it. Yes I'm an overthinking perfectionist, so I even wanted to do THAT the right way.

Thankfully, the decision I did make was to try something else first. I decided since I was emotionally ready for my life to be over, I would make myself well again the natural way, or I would die trying.

My focus shifted to wellness and yet I was ready for the consequence of death if I failed. The life of autoimmune misery, lying in bed for days at a time, missing out on everything, was not the one I wanted to live anymore.

Whenever I make up my mind, that's it. I go for it with all I've got. I knew my current state of being was not something I wanted to endure for the next forty-some years, if I could make it that long.

Even if you don't feel radically disciplined, you'll learn how you can work on mastering that skill, and start feeling like you are getting your life back.

The truth is your health has got nothing
to do with luck.

You aren't unlucky —
you just haven't been given the
right key to unlock the right toolbox until now.

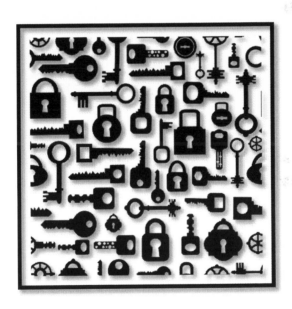

NOTES

CHAPTER THREE

The Trifecta

Change is unfamiliar. It might feel scary.
The relief comes from knowing your strength is
already inside you. You just need to find your "why."

They say once you know better you can do better, and having the knowledge to know how autoimmune illness starts means you can do better to live your best life in key areas going forward. I focus not just on health but also a little on finances too, since way too many autoimmune warriors, just like you, have been forced to cut back or completely stop working at some point because of illness. It breaks my heart, as I know the place you're at. If you ever dreamed of being self-employed, my guess is you stopped dreaming when you got sick. Or maybe your dream is to move up the ladder in your corporate career, but being this sick probably means it's off the table now. (It isn't!) And in the depths of this illness, it's almost impossible to afford basic costs of living or drive a safer vehicle, let alone dream about traveling, owning a home, or seeing your kids grow up and have families of their own.

I was at the end of my rope, and I hope you never get to that point. Or maybe we all need to get to that feeling of absolute desperation before we really dig our heels in and are nudged — no, *forced* — to do something differently. Maybe it's the anguish and despair that causes us to want to do more than just survive, but find a way to thrive again. I missed thriving. I missed feeling fully alive, and missed feeling excited about life. I wanted a future I could look forward to, not one in a wheelchair and on an organ transplant list like so many others with autoimmune illness face. I know you want a future you can look forward to as well. But what does it look like right now, if you do nothing to turn your health around?

There are three components that commonly set off autoimmune illness in almost everyone who has one; I refer to this deadly combination as the perfect storm; a *trifecta*.

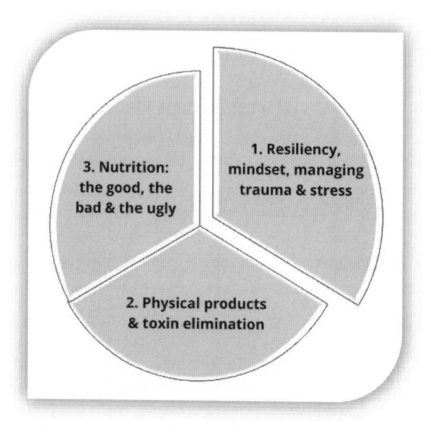

These three things led to my health crisis, and yet paradoxically, were also exactly how I got my life back again.

We are about to analyze the trifecta in detail. Get ready for a breakthrough — maybe several.

You will learn about toxins, what to eat, what not to eat, what factors contribute to an unhealthy and a healthy mindset, as well as practical, tangible things you can do and avoid to benefit your autoimmune health.

You'll maybe even improve your financial wellness in the process. You'll gain confidence to make informed decisions that affect every aspect of your life, and you'll love yourself enough to choose the best choices based on the outcomes you want to have. Most importantly, you'll know how to unlock your own ability to heal.

1. Mindset needs to be your first stepping stone on your path to wellness, but on a deeper level than just thinking positive thoughts. The definition of insanity is doing the same thing over and over and expecting a different result. After years of being in a victim mentality, stressed out about everything, wondering why I was hit with disease after disease, angry at the people who had hurt me, resentful towards the doctors who had brushed off my symptoms, wondering why everyone around me was having a better life than I was, thinking I didn't have enough money to live a healthier, happier life, wondering when I would die, and believing someone else needed to figure this out — I came to the realization that I needed to step up and take charge of my life and my recovery.

I had been stuck in a pinball machine, bouncing from doctor to doctor for several years before having this epiphany. I was finally so fed up with pretty much every aspect of my upside-down life that I decided I was willing to do whatever it took to be right-side up again. No one was going to do it for me, despite all my complaining. There was an energy shift in me; a new intentionality.

Instead of asking yourself, "Why is this happening to me?"
ask yourself, "What is this teaching me?"

Acknowledge that you didn't ask to be in this
position, and then, "What am I going to do about it?"

It wasn't that I haphazardly daydreamed things could be different. There is a vibrational energy in us and when you intentionally focus on something for your life, to the point you FEEL it absolutely WILL happen, this is the turning point. Visualizing your healthy life in great detail is a very powerful tool. I even went so far as to tell my family doctor my goal, and it wasn't to ask for his guidance — I told him I would make myself better. I know he didn't believe me, but that's how serious I was. I knew deep down if I didn't make these changes, I would very likely be miserable and unhappy for the rest of my days, however many I had left before death.

Systemic lupus and mixed connective tissue disease are scary. As are all the other autoimmune and metabolic diseases. Even though it seems normal these days to have a low thyroid because of lifestyle and the trifecta of toxins, people die from autoimmune conditions every day. None of this should ever seem normal. I didn't want that to be my story, and I don't want it to be yours. Now, changing your mindset is a choice, yet there are reasons many people struggle with doing so.

Trauma is one of the biggest hurdles. Some people don't know they've had trauma, or don't remember the specifics because the brain locks away bad memories as a protective survival mechanism. Some people may know their trauma but be unwilling to explore it and dig deep because of how painful and stressful it is to think about. The irony is that the trauma is a contributing factor to the chronic stress and physical pain you're now having to endure. Exploring your past experiences with the help of a professional and/or guided techniques can help release it.

2. Physical products and eliminating toxins: I used to think people who used all natural stuff and complained about grocery-store deodorant were ridiculous. Why would companies be legally allowed to sell things that were harmful?

I didn't believe it was a problem until I was at my breaking point with the side effects of all the prescriptions I was taking, began looking into what else was an option, and learned why people use natural products in the first place.

Toxin accumulation is one of the most significant tangible threats the human body faces today. Our body absorbs everything we put on our skin, in our hair, on our eyelashes, lips and face, and everything we breathe in. It all ends up in our bloodstream, either through absorption or inhalation. Don't think you don't expose yourself to toxins. Dryer sheets are one of the most toxic household products. They leave a hormone-altering residue on all your clothing and sheets that touches your skin day and night, 24 hours a day, 7 days a week, 365 days a year. Every single product in your home is either 100% natural, or is toxic. If it isn't made from plants and minerals, your liver and kidneys work overtime to filter it out. Environmental toxins as well as toxins in our food supply can interfere with our body systems and cause us to have anxiety and depression symptoms. Pesticides and fungus are toxins to the body, and are in so many things we eat on a daily basis.

Not only are you about to embark on a learning expedition about your body and how it reacts to a lifetime of using synthetic products, you'll learn what products are safe.

3. Nutrition is the fuel for our body, and yet so many people have no idea of how to do this properly. They wait for their family physician to explain it. Dementia, Alzheimer's, depression and anxiety are inflammatory disorders, and many foods in the standard North American diet trigger inflammation. Pesticides in the world's food supply are a huge health crisis and alarmingly there are over 1,000 pesticides used around the world. The Government of Canada (Canada.ca) and the World Health Organization (WHO.int) claim "pesticides play an important role in making sure there is enough food for everyone, by protecting crops from pests like insects, weeds and fungal diseases." The WHO also acknowledges pesticides are potentially toxic to humans and can have adverse health effects. And yet they are in most modern food production, unless you are eating food labeled as organic.

Keep the trifecta in your mind as you go through each of the chapters in this book. Every topic I talk about links to the trifecta in one way or another. Print out the graphic and hang it on your fridge or mirror if that would be helpful. As an additional resource to this book, I have included a printable version of it for you on my website. Please see the back page of this book for the specific URL address.

By focusing on the trifecta piece by piece and learning what contributes to autoimmune illness and what you can do about it, you can change your physical health, your mental health, your financial future, and your vibrational energy. Even the longest or most difficult journeys are achieved like any other — by taking one step at a time.

The biggest transformations come from doing small things daily. You will get the results by focusing on the process.

It's time now to do something different if you want something different. When you are truly living a high-vibin' life, illness and financial hardship aren't on your radar anymore.

NOTES

CHAPTER FOUR

Trauma and the Nervous System

We may be changed by what happens to us,
yet we can control what it means for us.

The understanding and treatment of trauma has significantly evolved as doctors and researchers continue to learn about trauma's effect on the brain and body. In decades past, trauma survivors were often misdiagnosed with depression, substance abuse, or mood disorders — symptoms of the underlying issue.

Traumatic experiences at any age can rewire the brain to be on constant high alert for danger. The event can be so overwhelming at the time that part of the brain turns off while the "survival" area of the brain takes over. The experience is not processed or stored away appropriately "in the past" as with other life situations, and therefore the event is seemingly never over. A person can unfortunately continue to experience the trauma event as if it's happening again, over and over, triggered by even the smallest thing.

If you aren't convinced yet that emotions have connections to your body, just think about what happens when you look at a picture or video of a snake or large spider, watch a video of a roller coaster ride, imagine yourself speaking in front of a crowd, or plan to drive yourself to an appointment in an unfamiliar city. Chances are just reading this passage and thinking about these things (let alone seeing the images or the real thing) has caused some butterflies in your stomach or caused your armpits to start feeling sweaty. The thought led to an emotion, which caused a physiological response.

Our nervous system has two states: sympathetic and parasympathetic. We were designed to live mostly in a parasympathetic state of contentment, relaxation, and peace — and to thrive in life. Our sympathetic state was necessary for survival — as a temporary measure to get us out of harm's way in a hurry so we could return to our parasympathetic, thriving way of being. This is the ideal, but is no longer the norm for a vast segment of the population.

Modern-day stress occurs when life events are more than we can cope with. It can be short-term stress like right before a job interview, or chronic stress as when living with or working with people who continually gaslight you, or if you are looking after an aging or terminally ill parent with no relief in sight, or if you've been diagnosed with a significant illness. We tend to not think of stress and trauma as the same, but they actually elicit similar physiological responses inside our bodies.

When you experience fear, stress or trauma at any age, the reaction starts in your amygdala, the part of your brain that perceives fear. These experiences could be related to an accident, or abuse, abandonment, scary situations, a shocking health diagnosis or other medical-related traumatic situation (yours or if you witness someone else's), or perceived imminent danger. The amygdala is the starting point for a domino effect involving the hypothalamus-pituitary-adrenal (HPA) axis, which triggers the stress response.

Your body's sympathetic nervous system goes into "fight-or-flight" mode. You need this physiological reaction because it keeps you alive in times of physical danger so you can fight off attackers or run away. Another response, freeze mode, is a self-preservation technique often experienced by victims who have survived assault when fighting could make it worse and fleeing isn't physically possible.

During the body's normal stress response, your hormones help regulate (increase or decrease) your blood sugar, blood pressure, metabolism, sleep, reproduction, digestion, sensory perception, hunger, fear, stress response, movement, sexual development, growth, and more. Your body goes into survival mode and the functions required for imminent survival are kicked into high gear while the functions for regular everyday life are put on hold.

The adrenal glands secrete the hormone adrenaline (epinephrine), which rapidly responds to stress by increasing your heart rate and rushing blood away from things like digestion, and to the muscles and brain. It also spikes your blood sugar level by helping convert glycogen to glucose in the liver. Adrenaline causes quicker breathing and increased heart rate, gorging the muscles with enough blood to make them as powerful as they can be so you can run for your life. Survival is the only goal. All other bodily functions are impaired in a state of flight or flight. This entire cascade of events in your body is extremely beneficial for keeping you alive.

Ideally, the threat is short-lived and would then be gone; your day would return to normal. Your muscles could relax and digestion and other regular bodily functions could resume. But in modern-day terms, we are often feeling "under attack"; our muscles are tense and we are stressed out almost all day long. This stress response was handy for our ancestors when trying to outrun a predator and fighting for our lives, but problems occur when the body doesn't know how to shut off the response, or isn't able to bring down the levels to normal again. In this revved-up state, the adrenal glands are continually producing excess adrenaline and cortisol so we can fight or flee, but most of us don't burn it off through physical movement. Instead, we internalize our stress, try to appear calm on the outside while we bury it down deep, and we pay the price with our physical and mental health at a later date.

Not only that, but cortisol impairs melatonin hormone production, and melatonin supports immune function and sleep. Meaning, your immune function and sleep are compromised when your body is experiencing this continual stress response. Sleep is a significant necessity for our health, and things can fall off the rails quickly when we are not getting adequate, deep, regenerative sleep.

> *Chronic stress is not a badge of honor.*
> *You can't be in a constant state of*
> *sympathetic response and expect*
> *a parasympathetic result.*

Finding a daily physical outlet for this built-up energy is important for the health of the adrenal glands, the overall endocrine system, and our gut health, which influence our physical and mental wellbeing. Past trauma and long-term stress can result in impaired communication between the immune system and the HPA axis, believed to be linked to many health issues including chronic fatigue (your body burns out from continual fight or flight responses), depression, metabolic conditions (such as diabetes, hypertension, obesity), and autoimmune disorders.

Chronic, profound fatigue can be a symptom of a malfunctioning liver, endocrine system, and/or the adrenal glands. You may have heard it called adrenal fatigue.

Just like pain, or any other symptom, adrenal fatigue is a message. A symptom is not "the" problem — it is a sign of something else going on.

Your body is exhausted and it's important to respond to its pleas for help.

The liver performs essential, life-sustaining functions for digestion and growth, and is critical for filtration to rid your body of toxic substances. Iron absorption is highly regulated by the liver, so if you have experienced unexplained anemia, it could be connected to poor liver health.

The liver is also associated with ruminating emotions of anger, resentment, hatred, sadness, frustration, irritability, bitterness and having a temperamental "short fuse." If you have had trauma in your life, and have not dealt with it or resolved it, you could be stuffing down these unresolved negative emotions and they may be contributing to your declining health. It would be worthwhile to explore this as a possible reason for your ill health, especially if all other factors (you eat a clean diet, get plenty of exercise, have detoxed your lifestyle) seem to be indicating you should be in peak health but aren't.

I was under severe stress in my career and my home life during the years I was at a breaking point with my health. The two situations seemed unrelated to me at the time, just a coincidence, but looking back, the correlation makes perfect sense.

Another form of trauma can be physical. Head injuries can occur from falls, physical abuse, car accidents, or sports. Concussion injuries are common in many sports, from contact and team sports to wake boarding and horseback riding. I got a concussion from a big wipe-out while wakeboarding a couple of summers before I got H1N1. I didn't know people should wear helmets for water sports. I mean, it's water. But it sure hurt when I tried to learn how to do a simple 180-degree switch and somehow ended up hitting the water headfirst, while still hanging onto to the tow rope.

Have you ever been in a motor vehicle / motorcycle / ATV accident where you hit your head? It might seem unrelated that someone who experienced a head injury in childhood or early adulthood could have endocrine issues in later years, yet when you look at where each of the glands are, and realize the pituitary, amygdala and hypothalamus are in the skull, it becomes glaringly obvious how an endocrine system malfunction can be caused from physical trauma. If the glands are damaged and not functioning properly, a "domino effect" malfunction and subsequent hormone imbalance can occur.

I know way too many women who are on thyroid medication for a low-functioning thyroid gland. I bet you do too. The hormone known as T3 is like gas for the car — you need it to be able to go anywhere. A sluggish thyroid also means sluggish digestion and sluggish nutrient absorption.

Prescriptions manually adjust the hormone levels but don't fix the underlying cause, which will continue to fester like mine did. In fact, I only recently discovered that the prescription I was on only adjusts the T4 hormone, and that a large percentage of people with hypothyroidism have Hashimoto's disease (also known as Hashimoto's thyroiditis), one of the most common autoimmune disorders. I was never told any of this by my doctors, and the thyroid tests I had done were only ever basic-level, not comprehensive, and without further investigation. According to the Thyroid Foundation of Canada, five times more women than men have hypothyroidism, and more women than men are affected by Hashimoto's, with a ratio of at least 10:1.

Millions and millions of women are struggling to manage their everyday life because of a malfunctioning endocrine system, and Western medicine is failing to look for causes. Men suffer from autoimmune illnesses too, but there is a significantly higher proportion of women affected. This may be due to more women than men being exposed to indoor air toxins from household cleaners, as well as the hundreds of endocrine disruptors in skin and hair products, makeup, and birth control pills. Plus, statistically, a higher number of girls and women are victims of trauma (sexual abuse and domestic violence). Girls also process trauma in different areas of the brain than boys do.

The powerlessness that comes from experiencing trauma can cause a response known as learned helplessness — which can turn into chronic lack of self-esteem, low motivation, giving up quickly, and believing you will fail, so you think, *"Why bother trying at all?"*

Please let me be crystal clear: I am not at all suggesting that trauma you experienced at the hands of another person was your fault. And as children, if that's when the trauma occurred, we do not have the emotional capacity and understanding to healthily process the event(s) ourselves, without professional counseling. In fact even as adults it can be very challenging to process these things on our own.

Trying to simply not think about it won't make it go away. Your body and your subconscious remember. We weren't responsible for the trauma happening to us, but as adults, it IS our responsibility to work on healing from it. No one else can do this for us.

Continuing to push yourself, going about your daily routine, and ignoring all the warning signs like flashing lights in your car's dashboard are ingredients in a recipe to get catastrophic results.

Your body is trying to communicate with you.
It needs help. You need to find balance for
your endocrine system immediately
and the sooner you start, the better.

Nine Foundational Steps:

Foundational Step 1:

Carrying around negative energy from the past impacts every area of your life: your health, relationships, ability to create wealth, your connectedness (to others and to a higher power, supreme being, or the universe), and your ability to be who you feel you were meant to be.

Every physical ailment has an emotional component. Many of us experienced some form of trauma early in life that can now be causing a physical symptom or multiple symptoms. If you have been the victim of trauma, it is really important to seek professional therapy with someone well-qualified, to learn healthy ways to understand and process your emotions, and begin to heal from your experience. Yes, you can heal from trauma; you don't just have to "cope" with it anymore.

As a self-help resource book, *The Body Keeps The Score: Brain, Mind, and Body in the Healing of Trauma* is a worthwhile read. (Written by renowned trauma expert, psychiatrist Bessel van der Kolk, M.D.)

Cultivating new behaviors and thought patterns
will strengthen and expand your resilience —
and resiliency is life changing.

Foundational Step 2:

Consider the potential outcomes and consequences of getting better vs. not. One of my favorite business tools is called the S.W.O.T. analysis: a strategic planning technique which examines strengths, weaknesses, opportunities, and threats. (See the chart on the following page. Download the printable version of the S.W.O.T. analysis from my website to use as a worksheet — see the back page of this book for the URL address.)

Not only is the S.W.O.T. analysis a helpful way to build resilience in a business, it's an extremely beneficial exercise to perform in our personal lives, too. Identifying our own weaknesses (in our mindset, our health, our finances, and our relationships) as well as potential threats (risks to our health, finances, and enjoyment of life) can help us come up with creative solutions. Threats (real or perceived) cause our stress response to fire up.

Planning how to improve or work around our weaker areas and mitigate threats helps reduce the stress of the "unknown." *Calmness in the storm* comes from knowing in advance what we can do in any given situation, and following through will feel easier if and when the situation arises. Being aware of our strengths and identifying opportunities encourages clarity for moving forward, builds self-confidence, and generates excitement about the future.

	Helpful	Harmful
Internal	*Strengths*	*Weaknesses*
External	*Opportunities*	*Threats*

Reflect on your health, relationships, finances, and enjoyment of life. What are your (internal) personal strengths you can draw on or that others often come to you for guidance about?

What are your (internal) weaknesses and areas you know you need to improve? What opportunities have presented themselves to you recently? What can you do to create new opportunities for yourself? And consider some possible "threats" to your health, your relationships, and your finances that could be a result of choices you make, or don't make. Observe where most of your actionable changes are placed. Work on the easier ones first for some quick wins.

This may be the first time you've really thought about the "what ifs," and it may feel like a punch in the gut. Maybe this is exactly what you need right now to prompt you to get intentional. At least some of what I cover in this book is information you already know. But for some reason you've held back. Why is that?

Many of us (possibly most?) have limiting beliefs. If yours relate to your belief in your ability to be healthy or successful, it could be one reason you give up easily or frequently fall into a self-sabotage pattern.

If you do nothing, what will your life look like in six months? In a year? In five years?

This is emotionally hard work, I get it. Honestly, without a burning desire within you to really do this, and without doing some emotional excavating, the chances are high you will put this book down and only do a few things or none at all. If simply feeling better was an ideal motivator, the world would be full of millions more healthy people with very few health issues. Think of the number of times you knew eating or drinking something would make your stomach ache, or give you a headache, and you ate or drank it anyway. Think of the number of times you procrastinated on working out or going for a walk, knowing it makes you feel good, but you continually allowed other priorities to move up to the top of the list.

Healing from an autoimmune malfunction requires
a major shift in everything you do and in how you think.
Get ready to do the work, and you'll reap
the benefits 100 times over.

Foundational Step 3:

Identify what motivates you. In chapter two, I talked about my own "radical discipline" and wondered if it was the x-factor in what propelled me forward on my path to wellness. But in my research of other people who have also overcome challenging autoimmune conditions, they didn't all have that characteristic. What they DID have, however, was commitment, and it was for their own personal reasons, based on their core values.

This commitment, which for me shows up as radical discipline, is what convinces you to do the hard stuff even when you don't want to. For some people health is a core value, whereas for others being healthy allows them to realize other core values and life goals. One of my core values is financial security, and while it doesn't seem related to making better health choices, at one time I was so sick I couldn't work or earn a living. I also advocate (for myself and others) home ownership rather than renting, because it offers the owner future financial security. Not being able to work makes it hard to make mortgage payments, or rent payments for that matter. It feels scary and stressful to be worried about money all the time.

While at first glance a core value might not seem related to your wellness, give yourself time to reflect on why you really want to feel better. What will wellness give you in your life? Your brilliant, creative mind will connect the dots sooner than you might think.

You'll have more opportunity to explore this idea further in the next chapter.

Foundational Step 4:

Do daily mindset practices. Journaling and vision boards are helpful to put your thoughts into words and pictures. Grab yourself a notebook or two. Set a reminder in your phone or calendar to journal your innermost thoughts every day, such as why you react to the things you react to, and again, really dig deep. Release pent-up feelings through writing. Don't let your fear or embarrassment prevent you from journaling your deepest thoughts and greatest epiphanies. Create and say affirmations.

Speak positively about yourself even if at first you don't believe it, and speak positively about others. Add words of inspiration to your vision board, or write encouraging notes to yourself on your bathroom mirror.

Foundational Step 5:

Set boundaries for yourself to stop meddling in other people's lives and set boundaries for those meddling in yours. A lack of boundaries, or constantly thinking you need to fix everyone else's issues, can quickly land you smack dab in the middle of other peoples' negative energy and complex life situations. This can cause unlimited amounts of stress in your life (and theirs) and can trigger your fight or flight response.

My friend Lauren da Silva is a boundaries boss, and if you struggle with boundaries, her book titled *A Heart-Centered Woman's Guide to Healthy Boundaries* is a must-read. She's also the friend who helped me embrace the idea of my radical discipline as the superpower that it is, rather than thinking of it as an annoyance to other people. When we can't see the forest for the trees, sometimes having a conversation with someone we trust can result in profound changes to our self-perception.

Make the decision that everyone (you included) will focus on their own stuff from now on. Everyone is capable of being responsible for their own life (children of course need more guidance than adults but this can come incrementally). Setting boundaries helps you avoid drama and keeps you in a more focused, positive mindset rather than being pulled in different directions that aren't meant for you.

Let everyone else make their own decisions (unless they directly ask for your help) and let yourself make your own decisions for you. This goes for in-person as well as on social media. If social media tends to get you riled up, take a break or limit your online time to short periods, at least for the time being. Besides, you're going to be busy getting better.

Foundational Step 6:

Do you ever eat or drink anything that makes you feel like you're suddenly nervous, with a racing heart and fluttery stomach? If you know caffeine, chocolate, sugar (in all its variants) or other ingredients are contributing to your stress-fear response (or keeping you awake at night), try eliminating them from your diet for a couple of weeks.

This conscious choice in avoiding trigger foods can help you feel "unflappable" and you'll be more resilient to handle life's day-to-day stresses. Stress is often a trigger for diarrhea, upset stomach, heartburn, and indigestion, so avoiding these ingredients can help you feel more at ease.

Foundational Step 7:

Your body needs to burn off excess adrenaline and cortisol. Daily exercise, ideally outdoors in fresh air, is critical to your mental and physical health. Set a reminder in your phone or calendar and don't let yourself come up with excuses as to why you can't. That's called self-sabotage. You choose your priorities. And this one is so important to be at the top of your to-do list.

Can you fit outdoor exercise into your existing day? Yes you can. Maybe you usually drive the kids to school or extra-curricular activities when you could walk there instead. Or maybe you spend an hour (or more) daily watching TV, YouTube or listening to podcasts and could listen to your favorite speakers on your smart phone as you go for a walk. Maybe you usually sit in the car while waiting for the kids to finish their extracurricular activities — hop out and get stretching. Walk around the outside of your building or around the block on your coffee and lunch breaks. Whatever your normal daily routine is, get creative! If there's a will, there's a way.

Foundational Step 8:

Yoga is a useful combination of exercise and becoming familiar with your breath, body and mind. Many people find it extremely helpful for strengthening their body while improving their ability to be present, and "in the moment." Being mindful about what is happening "now," in any given moment, can interrupt negative thought patterns connected to worry and overthinking. I use yoga DVDs and there are many online sessions for free or low costs if you aren't able (or don't want) to join in-person classes.

Foundational Step 9:

If you have an emotional wall or a block related to your health, money, self-worth, or success, it can be said a wall in one area of your life will be a wall in other areas of your life. You may be holding yourself back for some reason, consciously or unconsciously. Perhaps because of things that were said to you in childhood, or by someone you trusted who hurt you, you might not believe you are worthy of living your best life, or worthy of being successful, or worthy of being healthy. Or you might not believe you are capable of doing the things needed to change your lifestyle or habits.

Mindset work to explore your core values and limiting beliefs can be really helpful; and sometimes forgiveness can be the way forward.

Aromatherapy

Diffusing essential oils can be very beneficial to help release difficult, long-standing emotions and calm the stress-fear response without chemicals or pills. I like to use Lavender, Black Spruce, Cedarwood, Frankincense, or Cypress, and there are many others.

I also often rub a few drops of essential oils over my liver as well, to help process any negative emotions, support my parasympathetic nervous system, and help with filtration and digestion.

I highly recommend finding a certified AFT (Aroma Freedom Technique) practitioner to help guide you through a mindset session. I find the combination of inhaling essential oils with mindset work are extremely effective for stress relief which relaxes my entire body for the next few hours following each session. This relief does more than just allow me to feel good; it puts my body in a parasympathetic state of regeneration and repair. An AFT practitioner is ideal for personalized one-on-one mindset guidance, or you can look online for pre-recorded AFT sessions; many are free. Technology these days puts information at our fingertips — use it!

NOTES

CHAPTER FIVE

Creating Your Personal Matrix

Our values are determined by the source of our beliefs.
What are your fundamental beliefs and
do you know where they came from?

To achieve the goals you set, including your goal for better health, the goals must be in alignment with your identity and who you are. You might be wondering what on earth values have to do specifically with autoimmune health or feeling better. Without reflecting on and following your core values, you won't feel connected to, or in alignment with what you are doing. It will be hard to continue making healthier decisions if your actions don't really mean much to you or if they feel like a punishment. Being intentional about the food you eat, how much water you drink, whether you exercise, what products you use, and what you think about will all contribute to your health (or your illness).

Your core values will be your motivators on days you feel like your willpower is waning.

Do you value financial independence as one of your core values? Have you been unable to work, and want to start earning income again? Returning to work in itself is not likely your true motivator — it's the freedom and relief financial security brings. Having money allows you to pay all your bills whenever they come; no more stressing about how to pay them. So that would be the motivator, not the job itself. For others, exploring the world is the "prize." Travel requires health, stamina and the financial means. Do you wish you had more energy to play with your young grandchild? Why? (I mean, apart from the fact you love him or her, which of your core values is represented by spending time together?) Bonding with him or her, and sharing your values and beliefs as they grow up? Making new memories like you had (or perhaps missed out on) as a child with your grandparent? Giving them connection to their generational roots like you did (or perhaps didn't) as a child?

Often our core values are from our fundamental beliefs about the need to feel safe and secure: personal safety, financial security, love, and a sense of belonging in family or community are linked to this belief.

Certain core values may be rooted in positive early life experiences we found great joy in, or gained personal reward from, while other values become important to us because we were deeply hurt during childhood and developed the urge to protect ourselves and others. As one example, being given up for adoption could be a source of trauma and emotional pain in a child's life, and could lead an adoptee to detach from, or to highly value family, connectedness, and a sense of belonging. Everyone has different core values based on our unique life experiences and perspectives. Since our values are based on our beliefs, as we learn and grow we may also find our beliefs and values changing.

Dig deep, keep asking yourself why you want wellness, and then, when you think you have the answer, ask yourself why again. This process is relevant because once you discover these critical insights, it will feel significantly easier to be motivated to make and follow through with the day-to-day decisions that contribute towards your ultimate big goal.

Please don't skip this upcoming exercise, seriously.

Creating your own personalized matrix is the most critical component to your wellness journey.

ACTION: Grab a pen! Using the "core values" list on the following page, circle or write down the top ten values that are most important to you. These should be your guiding principles most relevant to you, that you try to live by, and that you also admire or respect in other people. The list of values and the matrix you'll be filling out are also available for printing on my website. Please see the back of this book for the URL website address.

From your list of ten, let's narrow it down. What are the **top four core values** that are most important to you and that you would be unwilling to give up?

Next, identify your **Superpower:** a long-standing characteristic or quality that makes you unique, and that you love helping others with too. If you're stuck for ideas, usually your close friends will know!

Your superpower is often related to (or might be the same as) your number one, non-negotiable core value — a must-have in your life, above all else. This means you could choose an additional core value for your matrix you'll be filling out on page 61 or your worksheet; your final list needs to consist of five words or phrases that you'll add into the boxes to complete the X.

Core Values

Accountability, adventure, athleticism / being fit and active, authenticity, balance, beauty, boldness, cleanliness, collaboration, community involvement, compassion, competency, consistency, courage / bravery / valor, creativity, credibility, dependability, determination, diversity, education / continuing education, empathy, enthusiasm, fairness, faith, fame, family connectedness, financial independence, friendships, fun, giving back, honesty, honor, humor, inclusiveness / sense of belonging, independence, innovation, integrity, justice, kindness, knowledge, love, loyalty, making a difference, optimism, passion, peace, perseverance, positivity, protecting animals, protecting the environment, reliability, respect, safety, service to others, speaking up for others, speaking up for yourself, spirituality, standing your ground, stability, teamwork, timeliness, trustworthiness, truth, vitality.

This is only a partial list to get your creative juices flowing. Feel free to look up values lists online and choose others if these don't feel quite right.

Make sure you have all five of the open squares in the matrix filled in on the following page (your cornerstone four core values and your superpower in the middle).

Additionally, having an open mind and willing approach to making lifestyle changes, being intentional about each of your choices from now on, and cultivating resiliency through the mindset work and stress-reduction techniques talked about throughout this book will complete your matrix.

	Intentionality	
Core Value		*Core Value*
Open Mind		**Resilience**
	Your Superpower	
	Willingness	
Core Value		*Core Value*

Now that all your squares are filled in, ask yourself why each of these core values are important to you. What made them become the traits you live by? You may want to write down your thoughts as they come.

Next, consider how each one connects specifically to your wellness journey and the future you most desire to have.

Reflecting on how *you* will be able to live *your* most amazing life when your health improves will directly impact every decision you make from this point forward.

Keep your core values and your superpower front and center in your mind as you go about your daily activities. Print out your matrix to put on the fridge, or if you're feeling crafty, create a decorative version of your matrix so you can refer to it as often as you'd like.

Every choice has the ability to support your core values and help you feel much more fulfilled about your life and purpose. Your intentional choices will help you heal, inside and out, and you'll begin to create the life you truly want.

This matrix you have just created will be the source for your own commitment and motivation (your own source of *discipline*) to stay the course on your healing journey.

NOTES

CHAPTER SIX

Forgiveness

Forgiveness is not about forgetting what they did.
It's about giving yourself peace.

I know this may feel repetitive, but it's important to dig deeper. Healing from autoimmune illness really starts from a foundation of emotional strength. Until you begin to understand and embrace the concepts of emotional intelligence, doing all the other practical, tangible things will just feel like "going through the motions." Emotional strength is very different from mindfulness and being radically disciplined. The point is not to turn a negative experience into a positive one. The focus is on feeling vulnerable, and sitting with those feelings with the purpose of allowing yourself to process them, understand them, acknowledge them, and no longer run from them.

When people bury strong emotions like shame, guilt and anger, they can develop destructive coping mechanisms like being controlling and criticizing; they may lack decision-making abilities because of self-doubt and low self-esteem, or become addicted to drugs, alcohol, sex, food, gambling, and more. Uncontrolled, strong emotional outbursts (crying, yelling, panic) can make daily life challenging. Normal, everyday things may trigger you, whereas they didn't before or don't trigger other people.

You are in control of your own health outcome. Self-reflection is an important aspect of emotional intelligence, and taking responsibility for how you got to this point in your life can be a gut-wrenching but necessary realization. Empowerment will come from taking responsibility for how you will move forward from here.

When I started having symptoms of chronic fatigue, joint pain, shortness of breath, and rashes, I kept going back to the doctors to "fix" me. I said things to my friends and family like, "They are the ones who went to school all those years; they need to figure this out!" I was frustrated. I was in blame mode. Honestly, I was really angry at the entire medical system but kept going back week in and week out because I didn't know I could do anything to make myself healthy again without a medical diagnosis and pills that would cure whatever it was.

I could have changed my diet then. I could have started learning about toxic overload then. I could have taken massive action to intentionally reduce my stress load by ending the relationship I was in, and by changing jobs. But I didn't. I waited. Because despite how hard it seemed to deal with those things, not dealing with them seemed less hard. As weird as it sounds, the familiarity of my day-to-day routine was comforting, even though I was unhealthy and unhappy.

I doubled my efforts on the toxins (unknowingly) by using more store-bought disinfectant sprays and wipes (thinking I needed to disinfect my home and myself to get better), and adding new prescriptions as each additional symptom reared its ugly head.

Many doctors didn't take my initial symptoms seriously, like the one who said I was "just depressed" and needed talk therapy. I had to have an appointment with our local mental health center because in order to qualify for missed work-wage loss I needed to do what the doctors advised. The psychiatrist talked to me for about fifteen minutes and then said there was no reason for me to be there. A month later I convinced a different doctor to do bloodwork and he discovered my thyroid function was very low. Even driving myself to doctor appointments was difficult (and risky) because I was exhausted and in a fog. I just wanted to sleep all the time and was literally sluggish because of a gland malfunction. It was still another year (eighteen months from my H1N1 episode and downward spiral from there) before I got referred to my rheumatologist and diagnosed with lupus.

I was relieved at getting some answers,
but by then the resentment of not being believed
was spilling out of me everywhere.

I used to be really angry at a lot of people. I held grudges against ex-partners who had wronged me, cheated on me, abused me, and caused me a great deal of stress, financial loss and heartbreak. I held a grudge for several years against a long-time close friend who stole from me. I held grudges against family members who had said insulting and hurtful things to me and those who had caused me to feel fear while I was a child. I held grudges against all the doctors who brushed me off when I was vulnerable and desperately asked them for help. When I was in the midst of the divorce case, another friend provided my ex with pictures from my Facebook account to use against me in court, making it appear like I was living the high life.

To this day I am still processing the lingering emotional effects of the toxic workplace I gave years of my life to. After additional organizational shuffling, when I was off on long-term sick leave, a manager removed all my medical information from my Human Resources file, then claimed there was no proof I was sick, and advised me I needed to return to working full time immediately. Because I was actually not well enough to work or keep up the battle, I faced an impossible choice. With fire in my belly, I wrote a scathing email as my official resignation. I have done lots of forgiving, but sometimes the memories creep back.

Life isn't always fair. We all have our own mountains to climb. Continuing to be angry, continuing to hold grudges, only hurts me. When you are holding tightly to anger, resentment and grudges, it only hurts you.

It's not easy to let go; I get it. I've been there. At first I didn't even think I wanted to let go of the anger, because it was familiar. Sometimes it almost felt good to contemplate revenge. But that's not actually a healthy response.

We can't find peace while dwelling on someone else's past wrongs or on situations that can't be undone.

Healing starts from within. Holding onto
past emotional pain is inflammatory.
It's in your best interest — your best health — to let it go.

When I'm angry, nervous or resentful, I feel it in my stomach. Our stress response to the memories and to the reliving of these traumatic moments will continually trigger excess adrenaline and cortisol production. The anger keeps us from enjoying life. Having a victim mindset (blaming

68

outward events or people) can prevent us from believing we can ever have the life we dream of.

Forgiving someone doesn't mean what they did is okay. It wasn't okay, and forgiving them doesn't make it okay. Forgiving the people in your life who have had a negative effect on you will be a huge relief. Forgiveness will cause a release of the tension and stress you are holding on to. It frees YOU of the anger and the emotional turmoil is it causing in your mind and body. You deserve to be free of those things.

Are you continuing to somehow attract stress, negativity, or traumatic situations into your life to this day? Forgiving yourself is another big step in acknowledging the self-sabotage and perhaps damaging role you have played in your own life. This may be a hard pill to swallow (pun intended) but you are now paying for it with your health. It's critically important to begin the healing process through forgiveness. Stress can be overwhelming, which literally wreaks havoc on your body. Sometimes we feel it right away, as if we were punched in the gut when someone wrongs us. Sometimes it is years later, after we have allowed the anger or frustration to fester, bit by bit, and have been holding onto our emotions all that time. Stress is a killer.

It's not enough to just agree you have stress in your life. It's time to deal with it, through setting boundaries and forgiving. As I've mentioned, one of the toxic relationships I dealt with when I first became really sick with lupus was my marital relationship. I was with him for over a decade. He was unfaithful, and manipulative. Gaslighting was a daily occurrence in our household, and I was unknowingly codependent. My feelings were determined by how he treated me (good and bad). If he was in a bad mood, his kids and I walked on eggshells. Our daily life seemed easier if we all made sure to "get along" and not disagree or "rain on his parade" in any way. Our household (with two children and two extended family members) revolved around him.

Two years after my lupus diagnosis I was pushed to the brink in our relationship when an incident of family violence took place and I had to call the police. I finally felt forced to make the decision to leave, and I could use the incident as my justification. I continued holding a grudge for a long time for what had transpired during our relationship as well as the continual threats, gaslighting and debilitating stress he caused me in the two years after we split up.

I have come to realize I didn't need a reason to leave, although I had a lot of reasons to choose from. I chose time after time to ignore them, until the incident was so violent I finally reached my tipping point. If you are in a similar type of relationship, or any relationship you don't want to be in for that matter, you don't need a reason to leave. You can choose to just go.

It took me a long time to forgive him because I thought that meant everything he had done was okay or that I accepted his behavior. As my friend Meggan Larson says in her book called *The Truth About Forgiveness*, forgiveness isn't for the other person. It's for you. They don't even need to know, and you don't ever need to tell them. Forgiving everyone in your life who has caused you hurt or harm is freeing and can unlock many emotional blockages.

I have also had to forgive myself for not seeing his behavioral warning signs much earlier; and even when I did see them, I have had to forgive me for allowing myself to be disrespected and emotionally abused for so many years before I drew the line in the sand.

What stress are you allowing to continue in your day to day life? And what traumas are you holding on to deep within you? The accumulation of wear and tear on your body and mind are like a concrete block tied to your ankle. You are stuck. You can't go anywhere.

I am showing you how to change your mind to change your outcome. I know this is hard. It might be the hardest thing you've ever had to do. But you'll have a much harder life if you stay stuck in an illness and victim mentality, bouncing around in the pinball machine.

Action steps you can start today:

Writing helps you get your thoughts out of your head without having confrontational conversations with people you may not want in your life. It's a way to safely explore your feelings, without consequence, and you can choose to keep, shred or burn what you've written. When you are ready, find a quiet place, and open your journal.

Make a list of people to forgive (focus on just one at a time). Write out your feelings, your *forgivenesses* (if this wasn't already a word, it is now), and your deepest desires for a better, healthier, fulfilled, content life going forward.

Block out time in your calendar and set a reminder on your phone or in your daily planner to work on forgiveness for 15-30 minutes. As you practice this skillset and get more comfortable in this space, you may find your list of people grows, and you'll also get faster at the forgiving process.

You can choose how to say it, but if you are needing some help with the words, a good script to start with is, "I forgive _____ (name) for _____ (what they did and how they hurt me)." If you are forgiving yourself, put your name in there and what role you played in hurting yourself or someone else.

Say your script over and over until you FEEL you believe it and truly feel you have forgiven them. In many cases this brings a flood of emotions, tears. Don't push those down — this is really important to let yourself feel and experience the release of these pent-up emotions that have been inside for so long.

Forgiving yourself is just as important. I know you're going to want to point out that you couldn't possibly have known _____, or have foreseen the consequences which resulted in _____.

Or there may be situations you look back at, and in all honesty think, yes, I can see that I did add fuel to the fire, or I did say some hurtful things, or told some lies because I was acting in fear. That's okay. This isn't about blame. Don't blame yourself. Forgive yourself.

Aromatherapy

- Geranium essential oil can help release negative memories, and encourage peace within the body.

- Lavender essential oil is calming, balancing, and can help put the body into a relaxed, peaceful, parasympathetic state.

- Frankincense essential oil can help peel off the layers of anxiety and depression from holding onto resentment.

NOTES

CHAPTER SEVEN

Mindset and Manifesting

There is always something to be grateful for,
no matter how small or how insignificant it
might seem to someone else. I bet you
have accomplished a lot in your life.
Probably against all odds.

Your own language often comes from what you were told or how you were made to feel as a child. It affects your view of yourself, your capabilities and your expectations of yourself and others. I have, and you probably have too, struggled through trauma on some level in our childhoods and adult lives, inflicted upon us by someone else. Whether it was neglect, emotional abuse, verbal abuse, physical abuse, sexual abuse, long hours alone as a "latch-key kid," or being ostracized by adults or peers, the negativity, judgement, and feelings of being on your own are detrimental to your self-perception. Even in adulthood, it might feel like you can't let go of the belief that the world is a mean, scary place.

It's so important to be mindful of your thoughts and words. I had gotten to a point in my health that I was fed up with my state of being, yet re-affirmed it to myself continually by saying things like, "I'm tired," or, "This day has gone to shit," even if it was still early morning and all I had done was spill my coffee on the floor. Dwelling on things that aren't how you would like them to be seem to make them bigger or happen more

75

frequently. Also, my tiredness at any given moment is not who I am. I may *feel* tired sometimes, but it's not who *I am*. Yes, the words matter.

I was resentful towards a lot of people, which I constantly felt in my stomach. I felt hopeless and confused about my health. I was worried sick (isn't that an interesting saying?) about my financial future. I complained about my job (up until I lost it), complained about my pain level, my random symptoms that seemed to make no sense, and what everyone around me was and wasn't doing that annoyed me.

Are you letting even the smallest things, or your words, cause thoughts that will manifest your future outcome?

The saying, "Be careful what you wish for" is such an intriguing phrase because of how powerful manifestation can be. The universe is always listening. I had often wished I didn't have my job because of the stress and trauma it was causing me. Then in mid 2016 suddenly I was in shock to have lost it. The universe picked up on my energy and the fact that I wanted to be free from that workplace.

Only a few weeks later, I was really worried about where to get money and had my mind on an opportunity for which I needed a lump sum. I had no source of income at the time but could not let go of the feeling I really, really needed to find a way to make this opportunity happen. I went to pick up my boyfriend Mike at work one afternoon and was in deep thought while stopped at a construction site when I was rear-ended by a large delivery van traveling at full speed, and then launched into a vehicle in front of me.

My injuries included partially separated shoulders, whiplash, and a hole in my retina from the force of the rear and front impacts. Mike's truck, which I was driving, was written off and my recovery included months of physiotherapy, massage and chiropractic treatments. The lump sum insurance settlement I later received helped fund the opportunity I had been thinking about that week. Believe me, I am NOT recommending getting in accidents as a financial strategy — it was a painful healing process. My point is be VERY careful about where your thoughts go and what you are manifesting for your life.

I am a huge fan of the film called *The Secret*. (If you prefer reading to watching a video, there is also a book.) It took me a couple of years to understand the message, which I think is because there was no mention of how to implement this technique. I was looking for an obvious answer, which there wasn't. It's somewhat ambiguous. However, once I started wrapping my brain around the concept, it was a lightbulb moment.

Do I believe just sitting thinking of a better
life will drop one in my lap? No.

To me, the law of attraction means if we
truly and deeply believe, AND if we start taking
steps towards reaching what we are striving for,
AND if we can just get out of our own way with our
limiting beliefs, we can do, have, or experience
whatever we put our mind to.
Another trifecta.

How to get into the right mindset:

Start telling yourself every day you are worthy and deserving of positive outcomes. When I first started doing this, it felt silly and untrue. Do it anyway, even if it takes a while to believe what you are telling yourself. Some of the affirmations I use (and have written on sticky notes beside my computer so I am reminded of them daily) are:

"I am worthy of feeling happiness."
"I am creative."
"I have my value now."
"I am making better choices for my health."
"I am making better choices for my financial future."
"I am in control of my health."
"I am in control of my finances."
"My health is my choice — I choose my health."
"I choose to eat wholesome food today to fuel my body and thrive."
"I am standing strong; I am healing."

Even if at first you don't "feel the feels," use these affirmations anyway. Your subconscious is soaking up every single word. Your own positive words to yourself will lead to dramatic breakthroughs in your relationships, your career, your mental and physical health, your finances, your creativity, and your children's lives (when they, too, learn the power of positive thinking and turning around their self-sabotage).

If after giving this a good try you still aren't believing yourself or your affirmations, you can add in an evidence step. I was introduced to this concept by my friend Dawn Shannon, and it not only changed the way I think about affirmations, but improved my results as well. Add the word "because" after the affirmation statement and give yourself the reason why you are in control of your health or your finances, why you deserve to have your happiness, or the reason why you are creative. Providing this *evidence* to yourself helps plant the idea more firmly into your subconscious and will help your self-esteem and motivation flourish.

You can also use affirmations that implicitly reinforce your power of positive thinking towards specific goals in your life. The more specific you are, the more focus your brain will give to that area of your life. Write your desired goal in past tense as if it has already occurred and you have already achieved it. "I am so happy and grateful now that I have achieved my goal of _____" (whatever it is).

Your subconscious will believe it;
your confidence will grow; your
mind will begin to unlock new thoughts,
you'll be more aware and curious, and you'll
feel more open to new opportunities.

Lower stress levels are a key factor to our body's ability to regulate itself, and to raising our vibrational energy. There is a direct and immediate impact on how we feel. We begin feeling excited and energized. It's an upward spiral (spiraling in the right direction up and over the wellness line).

Combined with the power of positive thinking, studies on the power of kindness show when we're kind, and when we do little things to make someone's day, we end up feeling happier and our stress levels go down. When you feel good and you make others feel good, the universe feels your raised vibrational energy and you naturally attract greater abundance and opportunity into your life (including better health).

Aromatherapy

Essential oils that can help increase feelings of positivity include:

- Floral oils (Rose, Ylang Ylang, Geranium)
- Tree oils (Frankincense, Black Spruce)
- Citrus oils (Bergamot, Lemon, Lime, Tangerine, Orange, Jade Lemon).

Try one at a time, and when you find one that you enjoy and that makes you feel really good, use it often. Feeling good naturally raises your energy vibration, which I will go into more in the following chapter. This in turn can help improve your health.

NOTES

CHAPTER EIGHT

Finances and Money Mindset

*Abundance in health, friendships, family, money, and
everything else you could possibly desire is waiting
for you if you are truly open to manifesting it.*

All matter is made of energy. Sound, frequency and vibration can literally alter physical material matter, which can be used as significant healing methods for many illnesses. Stress, negative thoughts and worry are lower frequencies, while happiness, excitement and celebration are higher frequencies. You need to keep your vibrational frequency high in order to assist with healing, and as abstract as this concept may seem, there are tangible ways to do this. Even if you think vibrational healing is "woo-woo," do these things anyway.

Your health will play a big role in your financial security. If you have been unable to work due to poor health, looking at your money situation may be a painful process but the "head in the sand" mentality (avoidance) won't help. You will continue to worry and wonder. Remember, you are now on a journey to overall wellness and when you take control of every aspect of your life, a whole new world will open up for you. Facing your financial situation is important.

Paradoxically, your financial situation will also play a big role in your health. Stress doesn't allow for creativity or good vibes. Living on next to no income makes it more difficult to take good care of yourself. And one of the biggest sources of stress for individuals, couples and families is money. Fighting about finances is one of the main reasons couples end up drifting apart and eventually splitting up. Whether you have a spouse or not, chances are you have worried about money a lot in your life, especially once illness began to creep in.

Your money mindset is your set of beliefs (or limiting beliefs) about money. Your beliefs were likely formed in childhood, from hearing grown-up conversations, or being told what money means to the adults who were teaching you. Your young mind soaked in every word.

"Money doesn't grow on trees."
"Dirty money."
"Money is the root of all evil."
"We can't afford that."

Your beliefs shape what you think you can and can't do with money, how successful you will be, how much income you will make, how you spend your money, how much debt you are in (and why you are in it), how much money you give away, and how you invest what you've got.

Before learning about money mindset, my finances were like a yo-yo; a ridiculous cycle of debt, frustration and then an influx of money that I would be excited about and then manage to spend right away. I was always stressed about where to get money, and then when I had it, I was stressed about what to do with it.

A scarcity mindset is when you fear losing money, you are afraid you'll never have enough money, you think money is tight, you are stingy about tipping, you feel like you can't make enough money (or the amount you want), and you worry someday you may end up broke. Your actions and thoughts are coming from a place of lack.

Using negative words can be like putting up subconscious roadblocks, and creating excuses or putting every other priority first are ways to self-sabotage, making it hard to move forward in any aspect of your life.

Energy flows where intention goes, so
always focus on positivity and abundance.

Cultivate a mindset of abundance by practicing gratitude every day and being thankful for all that you already have. An "abundance mindset" is believing you'll always have more than you need, while being open to new possibilities that may present themselves. An abundance mindset is not spending recklessly like you have a license to print money. There's a significant difference.

Focus on positive things, intentionally choose to be genuinely happy for people you know who are doing well financially, write and say affirmations to help alter your mindset from scarcity to abundance, and stop making excuses about why money isn't in your life.

These mindset exercises will help you to overcome limiting beliefs, which will lead to a healthier, happier outlook. Having an open mind and positive view of money can also allow you to see new opportunities you may not have considered before.

Action steps you can start today:

Recognize Self-Sabotage:

Telling yourself you are too sick or too broke to do something will cause you to believe it to the core of your subconscious. You are lowering your vibrational frequency with negative self-talk and it's important to interrupt the thought pattern to stop the downward spiral.

On the other side of the self-sabotage coin from feeling broke is impulsive spending on things that almost never get you closer to any of your goals. This can cause you to feel shame hours or days later when the money is gone, and you have lost the "high" you felt initially. Be honest with yourself and acknowledge your habits. If you do all your shopping using electronic accounts, you'll easily be able to go back through the last three months of transactions and see if this applies to you. Compulsive spending, much like other addictions, is a coping mechanism to temporarily deal with stress, pain, negative emotions, or feeling unworthy. It feels good at the time, but soon afterwards it makes you feel worse, which exacerbates your low sense of self-worth.

Working through past trauma, forgiving, managing your stress, and working on your mindset can be very helpful techniques to stop your self-sabotage in its tracks.

Be aware of your words. There are lots of ways we talk using negative words about ourselves, even if we don't intend to. For example: "I'm not a good cook." "I can't figure this out." "I'm not good at x/y/z." "I don't know how to manage money." "I'm terrible with computers." "I'm bad with money." "Money makes people greedy and I don't want to be greedy." Your subconscious and the universe hear this loud and clear, and continue to confirm it for you. You will attract more negativity.

Even if you don't like something, which is fine (I mean, none of us likes everything), you can use positive language to re-direct the focus to what you DO like. "I love journaling my progress." "I find it helpful using jars to manage my money better." "I appreciate having clear strategies to follow." "I booked a call with a financial advisor so I can learn how to make my money work for me." Positivity increases the vibrational energy around you and keeps you living above the wellness line!

Using conscious language and cultivating a positive mindset will be extremely beneficial to your health and financial wellness. Don't allow yourself to wallow in gloom and worry and despair.

Use the power of visualization by closing your eyes and encouraging yourself to feel every detail of how good your life will be when you reach your health and financial goals. Not if. When.

Create a long-term vision:

Set clear intentions on exactly how much money you want to earn and by when; how much per month; how much per year. Even if you don't know how you will do it yet, dream big! And write down your goal so you can see it and start focusing on it.

Write down your current net monthly income, then minus 10% to go to savings. From what's left, write down all your monthly essential bills — housing, utilities, food, your fixed loan payments, etc. From there, what's left needs to be prioritized — where is the leftover money best spent on things to get you closer to your goals? Think about how you will you feel when you gift some to your favorite community group or charity that you align with. Good people do good things with money, giving feels good, and feeling good raises your vibrational energy.

Work on paying off your debts as soon as possible, starting with the highest interest rate first. No one needs three or four credit cards. If you need a credit card for booking things like flights or hotel rooms, keep one card, keep the credit limit low, and pay it off every month. If your card balance is too high for you to pay it off each month, you are living beyond your means, and it isn't sustainable. The universe won't bring you more money if you can't manage the money you've got. And the stress is affecting your health.

Take responsibility. Are you recognizing the messaging throughout this book? Stepping up to the plate and taking responsibility is important for your finances, your health, your relationships, and every other area of your life. Know where your finances are at, at all times. At least once a week, book yourself a recurring meeting to review all your finances: Write down all the income that came in this week or month, review the amount of debt you carry (ALL of it!), and assess your net worth (including assets). A client once talked to me about the amount of debt she was in, and left out the car payments because she deemed those as "necessary," which in her mind meant it wasn't a debt. As strange as it may sound, everyone has beliefs around money, and identifying your areas of weakness will turn you into a guru!

Whether you do this "money meeting" alone or with your spouse or kids is up to you, but having everyone on the same page makes everyone feel like you are in this together and working towards the same goals together. The first meeting might be half an hour, but after that might only need to be five or ten minutes. Knowing your financial situation, especially if your goal is to pay off debt quickly, helps give clarity to your spending urges the next time you might be tempted to buy something you don't really need. It can also help kids understand why they can't always have everything they ask for, and it can help them learn to prioritize their desires and goals, too.

Reflect on and be grateful for what you have. Avoid ogling what everyone else has. If you are constantly thinking about what you don't have, what you focus on gets bigger and you'll continue to struggle with money and the mindset of lack.

If you want some additional income, perhaps you have a hobby or a lane of genius you could turn into an income stream. The saying, "It takes money to make money" is a money myth and a limiting belief. Lots of people work from home with very little overhead, which can be ideal if you like the idea of flexibility and being your own boss. Even more importantly for autoimmune warriors, working in your own toxin-free home, on your own terms, and on your own schedule can be a pivotal choice if the alternative is a stressful, unhealthy work environment.

If you love the idea of passive income, which is helpful in times you may be unable to work, rental properties are one of my favorites. As a landlord, you provide needed housing (I always allow pets, and my tenants have been very appreciative of this), someone else is paying off the mortgage debt, and the asset value (and therefore your financial security) almost always goes up over the span of the mortgage amortization. Yes, there are years here and there with dips in real estate values, but over the long term, the trend pretty much everywhere has been upward. You would always have the option to sell the property if you ever needed to, or if it's important to you to leave an inheritance for your children or other loved ones after your eventual passing, it could be gifted to them through your estate.

Aromatherapy

Certain essential oils have properties that are linked to emotions and can help you rebuild your relationship with money.

Oils that can help cultivate an abundance mindset (on their own or as a combination in your diffuser or a roll-on) are:

- Orange (happy and uplifting)
- Frankincense (calming and grounding)
- Cinnamon (associated with love and prosperity)

NOTES

CHAPTER NINE

The Endocrine System

Rock bottom can be a hard reality,
and it's from this place — learning from either our own
experience or someone else's — that we become
most determined to change.

Are you feeling sick and tired? Chronically exhausted? Muscle weakness? Stomach pain? Low blood pressure? Depression? Brain fog? We have the same cells and tissues in our gut as our brain. Functional medicine experts on the leading edge of research are now referring to the gut as our *second brain*, and referring to brain fog and cognitive impairment as "leaky brain."

Have you been told your hormones are out of balance, or has a friend suggested "your adrenals are shot"? Now that you know about conscious language, you are probably realizing this is not an ideal way to describe anything to do with your body or health.

Adrenal fatigue isn't the cause. And neither is lupus, or a low thyroid, or any type of other similar disease or illness.

By definition, a disease is "a disorder of structure or function in a human, animal, or plant, especially one that produces specific signs or symptoms or that affects a specific location and is not simply a direct result of physical injury." *(Oxford Languages)*

93

The illness, disease or condition is not the cause of or reason for your symptoms. The illness, disease or condition is the name given to the group of symptoms that you happen to have. Humans love to label things. These are a way to give a name or identifier to a cluster of symptoms commonly found in many people. Often, diseases are named after a person who first had the symptoms, or from the region of the world where these symptoms were first discovered, or may have the name of the doctor or scientist who discovered the symptoms in a patient who was ill.

Most doctors agree there are around 80 conditions that are considered autoimmune in nature. Many say there are over 100 and some science leaders are now saying that number is closer to 200. These illnesses have something important in common: a malfunctioning endocrine system.

The endocrine system is a chemical messenger system inside your body that gives and receives "instructions" to and from the organs called glands. This entire system regulates body functions, and controls your emotions, thoughts, and processing. The glands of the endocrine system are the communication link between brain and body. If those are not communicating correctly with each other, no matter how healthy you think you are being, your body and mind will not function correctly.

In a visual sense, think of the glands as a neighborhood of houses, with trails and pathways connecting each of the households to the others. Hundreds of postal workers (our hormones) are busy throughout the neighborhood carrying mail (messages with instructions) to each of the houses, at the same time. It's a buzzing little community with a lot going on.

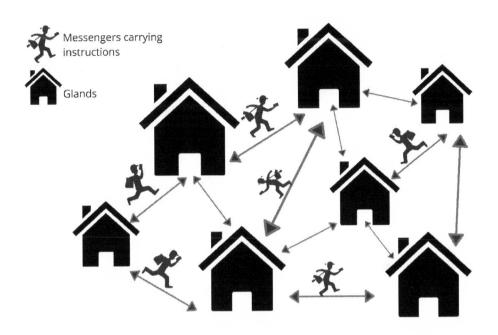

Messengers carrying instructions

Glands

These messages instruct each of the households (organs/glands) to do certain tasks and they keep the entire neighborhood (endocrine system) working collaboratively together.

This endocrine system chemical messenger system regulates everything from our sleep, behavior, excretion and metabolism to our growth, stress, mood, tissue function, digestion and more.

Visualize the postal messengers delivering mail telling each of the households what to do, when to do it, and how often to do it. Each household needs to also know what all the others are doing so the entire neighborhood can thrive together as a community.

But sometimes, early in our lives, some of these postal workers get interrupted, flustered and mix up the messages they deliver to each house. The mail and packages look similar, and the messengers are confused. The households are also confused because the packages look familiar but they can't quite decipher the instructions.

The households at first are often able to compensate and figure out what the right message or instruction should have been. Other times the households may perform the wrong task because of incorrect messaging instructions, but it happens so sporadically the rest of the neighborhood doesn't notice. Overall, the community is still humming along cohesively.

Over a longer period of time, these postal messengers continue to mix up the messages, deliver messages that don't make sense to the households, or not deliver them at all. Eventually, with each household not performing all of its required tasks for the good of the community, the neighborhood starts to go downhill.

The endocrine system is what triggers the glands to release hormones into the bloodstream so your organs and the rest of your body can function. This is why it's imperative this system functions at a peak level. You will die if it fully shuts down.

Adrenal fatigue is a sign your endocrine system is starting its downward spiral. Adrenal fatigue isn't the cause of your illness; your adrenal glands are malfunctioning for some underlying reason. Your "adrenal house" isn't receiving the proper instructions in the mail because of a disruption somewhere in the messenger service.

Lupus is also a sign of a malfunctioning
endocrine system. As is mixed connective tissue
disease. Irritable bowel syndrome. And all of the thyroid
diseases. And diabetes. And so many more.

Hopefully this is making sense so far and by now you are wondering what actually causes the messengers to get interrupted and flustered in the first place. After all, this seems to be where the neighborhood plan goes awry, right?

Critical thinking by digging deeper will increase your knowledge and propel you towards recovery rather than sitting back and thinking you're stuck with a messenger service that doesn't know what it's doing. Ask questions. Analyze. And always keep an open mind about learning. Science is continually evolving, and the more you read (from credible sources, of course), the more informed YOU will be about your body, your physical health, your mental health, and your options.

Don't rely on one doctor or one study. Get used to perusing Pub Med and other science-based articles frequently. Yes, they can be dry and boring sometimes, but I have had some epiphanies reading Pub Med articles! There are also some great functional medicine professionals who share information freely on social media.

Gradually you will begin absorbing the research and become much more confident about your knowledge and the decisions you make from here on in.

Root Causes of Autoimmune Disease

Many substances in the environment mimic or interfere with the body's hormones. They are known as endocrine disruptors. They interrupt, or disrupt, the messenger delivery system.

In simplistic terms, the endocrine system, which as you now know regulates so many of the body's everyday necessary functions, is also involved in regulating the immune response. This is the connection to autoimmune diseases.

Autoimmune diseases occur when the immune system perceives parts of the body as foreign and starts an immune response of "fighter cells" (white blood cells) to attack and eliminate them. If we continue to dig a little deeper, this process stems from the dysregulation of the endocrine system.

The job of white blood cells is to fight off dangerous viruses, bacteria and fungus that sometimes get inside our body, but with an autoimmune response these fighter cells recognize something isn't right, and they need to fight it off.

They begin to think healthy tissue is also foreign and needs to be attacked. This results in inflammation, which causes pain throughout the body including in tissues and joints, migraines, digestive issues, chronic fatigue, pelvic pain, mood disorders and other debilitating symptoms and additional diagnoses that those with autoimmune diseases often struggle with.

Reducing inflammation is an excellent focal point when deciding to make a change. Through my story, I'm showing you how I did it, and how you can too.

Have you got thyroid issues? Unexplained weight gain? Have you wondered why so many middle-aged women are on thyroid medication? Or why so many people are diagnosed with lupus and other autoimmune conditions these days? There is a common denominator linking us all, and it isn't genetics.

The CDC.gov (Center for Disease Control) website says, "The causes of SLE (lupus) are unknown, but are believed to be linked to environmental, genetic, and hormonal factors." Translation: environmental toxins, lifestyle (what we eat, how resilient we are against chronic stress), and hormone (endocrine) issues, which are also likely from toxins and stress. And this goes for so many more illnesses than systemic lupus. Many medical experts, as well as those who have turned their health around like I have, believe our genetics actually play an extremely limited role in our health trajectory.

When endocrine-disrupting chemicals block the connections between your hormones and their receptors, they "reprogram" the areas that govern metabolism, energy balance, and appetite, among other things. As one of numerous consequences, these chemicals change your sensitivity to glucose (sugar) and your metabolism of lipids (fatty acids). This predisposes you to gain weight, a very common complaint among middle-aged women. The endocrine disruptors that cause this have even been given a specific name — obesogens. If you have diabetes, you'll also want to look up the word diabetogen.

The endocrine disruptors mimicking our hormones are in many products we wouldn't necessarily think about, but they are also in things we ingest on purpose, such as synthetic estrogen (in birth control pills). Women often start using birth control (pills, injections, IUD) in their late teens while still growing and maturing. In many cases birth control is recommended by doctors to "regulate" a young woman's cycle or to help with PMS. Except that it's confusing to the endocrine system and interferes with the body's natural processes. If you are using birth control for anything other than contraception (as in, using birth control to try to fix other symptoms), you are experiencing a hormonal imbalance. Those symptoms are trying to tell you something.

My periods were irregular when I wasn't using birth control, so I appreciated having my body on a schedule. I was on birth control pills for over a decade thinking they were perfectly safe. I once tried the "depo" injection (injectable birth control) and had a terrible reaction to it. The skin on my face broke out in large, ugly, painful boils. When I went back to my doctor to ask if something could be done to counteract what was injected, he said I just needed to "wait it out." (The birth control product was effective for three months. It was a long, painful, self-conscious wait.)

The companies and the pharmaceutical industry tell us what is in their hormone pills and injections is "the same" as the stuff we make naturally, but it isn't. Our body knows something isn't quite right. The other households in the neighborhood are aware there's an imposter on the mail delivery team and they aren't sure what to do about it.

Other things that interfere with the messenger system are toxins that are in a wide variety of products we are told are safe — like plastic bottles, fire retardant used in the making of new furniture and moisture wicking clothing, food (pesticides and additives), children's toys, clothing, laundry detergents, dryer sheets, prescription medications, over-the-counter medications (pain relievers, anti-inflammatory pills and creams, muscle relaxers, muscle rubs, cough/cold/flu relief), and more.

The word "fragrance" on ingredients ranging from soaps and shampoos to candles, potpourri, laundry detergent, dryer sheets, scented markers for kids to color with, and even dog toys is a chemical concoction that is proprietary. Companies are legally allowed to hide what chemicals are in their products by using the word "fragrance" instead. It protects them from having to divulge their special recipe secrets.

Speaking of special recipes, many functional medicine doctors — doctors who look for root causes of illnesses — now believe many diseases once thought to be genetic are seen within family lines because generations pass down their traditional family recipes and lifestyle habits (often unhealthy ones). And not to be understated, patterns of abuse, trauma, and unhealthy coping mechanisms are also often repeated in each generation.

The chemical revolution's exponential growth over the past century has given us products we love and think we now wouldn't survive without, but the consequences of our constant exposure is dire — and it could be for decades to come. Our bodies are bombarded with hundreds of chemicals on a daily basis, from the day we are conceived in our mother's womb.

Everything a mother eats, drinks, breathes in, soaks in, and puts on her skin, affects her baby inside. Then for our entire lifetime from birth onward, we are continued to be exposed to synthetic, harmful toxins in our food and our environment, day in and day out. They are mostly filtered out, but not entirely. Bit by bit, there is a build-up of what can't be filtered, and this bioaccumulation is instead stored in our fat as a self-protection mechanism.

Eventually toxin overload, chronic stress, and unhealthy lifestyle choices can wreak havoc. The tipping point often happens in middle age, after a few decades of absorbing everything into our system from trauma to toxins, and the messenger system getting more and more disrupted and confused.

Don't be fooled by economical store products that claim to be "natural" because they have essential oils in them, or those with leafy green pictures on the front. Premium essential oils are too cost-prohibitive to add to cheap, mass-produced, synthetic cleaning products. Even the cleaning products with plants on their label are often distracting us from seeing the hormone-disrupting chemicals in the fine print.

Making products appear to be natural with a plant logo on the label and calling the product plant "based" because of one or two natural ingredients nestled among the toxins is called *greenwashing*. It's sneaky marketing to make you think the product is safe; meanwhile, these endocrine-disrupting products are contributing to your autoimmune malfunction.

Action steps you can start today:

If you are eating properly (whole foods, plant based, no meat/seafood/eggs, no dairy, no oils, no packaged meals), hydrating, exercising daily, but still not seeing and feeling significant health improvements, the next logical step is toxin elimination: a detox of your lifestyle.

Go through your kitchen, bathroom and laundry cupboards and grab every single package and bottle. Read the ingredients on every one of them. Toss out all the ones with the word "fragrance" on the label (remember, it does not mean the "smell." This is a clever marketing code word for lab-made chemical toxins.)

With any of the remaining ones, look up the ingredients online or use an app that rates how toxic and dangerous a product is.

Get in the habit of being disciplined about reading labels before bringing new products into your home. Write a reminder on your shopping list if you need to. Hopefully someday all the toxic, synthetic ingredients in everyday household products will be illegal, but in the meantime, we need to be sorting through what is and isn't contributing to autoimmune malfunction.

Give yourself more time in your shopping schedule because reading labels takes longer. Your health depends on it.

NOTES

CHAPTER TEN

Daily Dose of Toxins

Curiosity leads to learning, connecting and adapting.
These pave the road to resilience.

You can't always control if you get sick, but by understanding how your body works, what keeps it healthy and what can contribute to malfunctions, you have much more power than you think over your state of wellbeing. Once you have the knowledge, you can make evidence-based decisions with your health in mind.

You probably already know the immune system is your "defense" system, in place to protect you from pathogens and the development of disease. Immune cells are everywhere in the body. In your bone marrow. In your bloodstream. In your organs. They work hard to protect every inch of you from getting sick — the entire system works together to fight off invaders. In its natural state, the immune system is balanced and fully capable of doing its job, which is to keep you healthy. But the exposure we experience over our lifetimes, especially in today's era of chemicals and synthetics approved as legal and safe, is impairing our immune system's ability to do its job.

There is a misconception that people should always want to boost their immune system, so if you have been diagnosed with lupus, rheumatoid arthritis, Hashimoto's thyroiditis, or other overactive immune system issues, you may have been confused about why you feel so sick if your immune system is already hyperactive and appearing to be an overachiever. In fact this misconception causes many autoimmune warriors to be fearful of doing things that are commonly associated with "boosting" the immune system, like taking vitamins and eating more fruits and leafy greens. With autoimmune conditions, the immune system is not operating optimally, so it's important to aim for function and balance.

> *The easiest way to think about autoimmune disease*
> *is that it is a malfunction of the immune system*
> *because of a malfunction of the endocrine system.*

> *The malfunction is why you feel symptoms.*

I found that thinking of any of my diagnoses as a disease made me feel like it was terminal. But a malfunction sounds fixable, and perception is important for staying positive and focused on taking steps to get better.

You want to strive for rebalancing your body in every way possible, and one of the most important ways to do this is to reduce the toxin overload and let your body heal itself. Remember, too, that the benefits of processing past trauma and eliminating chronic stress can be life-changing.

If you have an autoimmune condition of any sort (including thyroid issues, psoriasis, diabetes, rheumatoid arthritis, lupus, mixed connective tissue disease, and others), very likely you have a toxin accumulation. Your body is finally saying "enough is enough" after a lifetime of trying to cope with the residue from dryer sheets and fragranced laundry soaps, synthetic ingredients in shampoos, conditioners, shaving cream, toothpaste, mouthwash, the fragrance (and smoke) in your evening candles, applying chemical make-up every morning, hairspray, hair gel, soaking your hands in blue dish soap they claim is gentle on animals but is full of stuff that actually isn't gentle, using disposable moist wipes, and spraying your doorknobs, handles, kitchen counters, cupboards, fridge, shower walls, toilet seat, sink and taps with highly toxic chemicals that you touch multiple times a day.

We also then add weird synthetic ingredients to our foods, such as pesticides in everything that isn't organic, aspartame, petroleum-derived products like food colorings, paraffin wax in chocolate, petro-chemicals in prescriptions and vitamins, shellac on candy coatings, and more. In the food industry, a petroleum-derived liquid called mineral oil is in a lot of packaged foods to keep them from going rancid.

Toxin accumulation is a really big deal. It happens ever so slowly, usually over decades. It's so gradual, it's hard to blame one product or one particular cause. And some people seem to be able to avoid illness while others become very sick (up to and including death from autoimmune disease).

Remember, autoimmune malfunctions are triggered by a deadly combination of toxin accumulation, chronic, profound stress, and a poor-quality, inflammatory diet.

In our early- to mid-thirties, our bodies often start to give off warning sirens. We've spent thirty-some years using and being around all kinds of products on our bodies and in our homes that have hundreds of chemicals in them. These toxins build up in our system little by little, ever so gradually; barely noticeable.

Sadly, by the late thirties and into the early forties, many women start experiencing some kind of health issue due to endocrine disruption. Most Western medical doctors often give pills as a first resort rather than trying anything natural or counseling their patients about what can affect endocrine system function.

In my case, after years of zapping pain and nerve-blocking medications for complex regional pain syndrome and then a hypothyroidism diagnosis, an even worse autoimmune condition came along: systemic lupus. Then another — mixed connective tissue disease. Western medical doctors simply prescribed pills to me, sent me to specialists for extra tests, and I was prescribed more pills. I'm sure you've probably experienced the same type of "treatment" that doesn't actually treat anything.

My experience was so awful that I wanted to write this book to help you avoid this train wreck if at all possible. There are SO MANY great things in life to experience, and I spent WAY too many months in bed feeling hopeless and depressed. I had pain that made me to want to amputate body parts and contemplate suicide. I was on pills causing damage to my health which I am still working on healing years later. My gut health, eye health, liver health, and brain health were all in jeopardy, not just from my inflammatory illnesses, but also from the prescriptions I was taking.

Simply stopping the pills didn't magically regenerate my body (and if you are wanting to change or reduce prescriptions you are on, please consult with a trusted medical professional. It can be very dangerous to simply stop taking medications).

Having a healthy body requires a lifestyle and mindset breakthrough. It's a new perception and a new way of living.

If you are suffering and frustrated, and your doctors (like some of mine) won't listen to you or say you are "just depressed," please hear me when I say you are NOT crazy, it's NOT all in your head, and you CAN do all kinds of things to take the pressure off your endocrine system to start the healing process.

I get it — not using dryer sheets ever again can be confusing. How on earth can a dryer sheet have anything to do with your health? The short answer is they are full of chemicals that confuse your hormones. They contribute to your body's mounting toxin accumulation with carcinogens, hazardous pollutants, and endocrine disruptors like benzene and acetaldehyde. You wear clothes all day with carcinogenic, toxic chemical residue on them, you rub the residue on your wet body with your fluffy terrycloth towel after a shower, and wrap yourself in your sheets all night long that have the residue on them too.

We are exposed 24 hours a day, 7 days a week, for our entire lives to dryer sheet residue, as just one of hundreds of ways we expose ourselves every day to endocrine-disrupting chemicals. Not to mention when you walk outside near a dryer vent and those hot chemicals are flowing out from peoples' houses throughout the neighborhood. Some of the chemicals in dryer sheets are the same as what comes out of a car exhaust pipe, and yet because these chemicals are masked with pretty-smelling perfumes, more people are worried about outdoor pollution than what's inside their own homes.

So much of what touches your skin goes straight INTO your bloodstream. Your skin is basically a big mouth — it is absorbent. Meaning, anything and everything you put on it goes into your body, and can begin a cascade of problems from a microbiome (gut bacteria) imbalance to inflammatory responses that lead to full-blown diseases!

And at the time of writing we are in the midst of a global pandemic where every single person is now being exposed to hand sanitizer in every store. Kids are all using hand sanitizers multiple times a day in daycares and schools. Have you seen on the news some of these products have been recalled because of their toxicity? The problem with a lot of the cheap, mass-produced sanitizers out there is they are loaded with synthetic and toxic ingredients you wouldn't want to feed to your body. Even some of the so-called "natural" ones still have fragrance on the label. Remember, "fragrance" is simply a brilliant marketing term to describe a toxic chemical concoction which soaks in and interferes with your hormone balance, your immune system, your gland and organ health, your skin, your gut health, and your brain health.

100% natural products are easy to buy or make and do not have any endocrine disruptors in them. The hand sanitizer I buy is made from denatured alcohol derived from Peppermint essential oil. I order it online and it is delivered to my door. It has no synthetic ingredients at all and smells delicious. How cool is that? Yes, it's a little more money than the endocrine-disrupting stuff but you need to stop choosing what's cheap and laden with chemicals over what's going to help restore your health. There should be no question about which one takes priority.

Do you see the connection now between autoimmune and skin disorders, headaches, hormone imbalances, and gut dysfunction to what products you've been using? When toxic ingredients get into your body through your lungs and skin they wreak havoc every which way.

The big take-away:

If you get nothing else out of reading this book, my #1 wish as a take-away for you would be to ditch the toxins in every area of your life.

Ditching the physical products is a quick win — it can be done cost-effectively and immediately, and will allow your body to stop being over-burdened day in and day out. You may even notice you start to feel better within a very short timeframe. Mindset work and "detoxing" your emotions takes longer, but the effects can be life-changing.

Detox your home. Go right now and gather up all your household cleaning and laundry products. Window/glass/mirror cleaner. Dryer sheets. Toilet bowl cleaner. Kitchen and bathroom sprays and scrubbing liquids. Air fresheners. Bleach. Remove the temptations and just toss them out now. White vinegar and baking soda are great toxin-free cleaners, and there are many essential oils with antiviral, antibacterial, and antifungal properties.

Use a 100% natural laundry soap or just some Epsom salts (not just plant "based" but all plants/minerals and nothing else, and no fragrance on the label). There are lots of great DIY recipes online for all natural laundry soap.

Got static in your clothes? Add a 1/4 cup of white vinegar to your laundry wash loads. You can also do an internet search for "non-toxic fabric softener." In our household, we haven't used dryer sheets or wool dryer balls in a few years — they honestly aren't necessary because vinegar prevents static. As for smelling nice, we put essential oils on our skin every single day, so it doesn't matter that our clothing isn't scented.

Detoxify your body by avoiding toxic ingredients, pesticides, and petrochemicals your body doesn't know what to do with.

Eat plants. Eat real, whole foods. The less packaged stuff you buy, and the less you eat out, the easier it gets to avoid these in your diet.

Find a functional medicine doctor or naturopath. They are your best resource for continuing to learn about how to heal your body naturally. They take a full history as your first or second appointment, because their interest is in getting to the bottom of what's happening in your body. The body malfunctions in mysterious ways, and they look for root causes.

As your endocrine system and stress hormones settle into a more balanced, healthy, parasympathetic state, you may notice you have an improved mood and less anxiousness. For those who have lived their life with perpetual worry and dread, it can be really eye-opening to experience what relaxation feels like without drugs or alcohol. And with some additional supports to help you process old traumas, it'll feel like a huge weight has been lifted of which you may not have even been consciously aware.

Your gut health is affected by not just diet alone — as you have now learned, products you use on your skin and in the air end up in your bloodstream by absorption and can contribute to poor gut health. Gut health also plays a key role in your mental health, so cleaning up all the toxins in every facet of your life can be life changing. Everything is connected.

Bonus: ditching toxins and switching to plant/mineral cleaners like white vinegar, lemon juice, baking soda, Epsom salts, castile soap, and antimicrobial essential oils actually costs less money than you are spending on your collection of various store-bought toxic household products.

NOTES

CHAPTER ELEVEN

The Wellness Line and Essential Oils

Much of your health is within your control.
Everything you do and think either adds
to your vitality, or takes away from it.

I was well on my way to wellness through improving my diet and managing my stress before I realized the effectiveness of essential oils. In fact, when my friend Megan Bailey first gave me some oils to try after my accident in 2016, I thought it was a funny concept that little bottles of plant juice could do anything for me at all. I tried a couple of them one time, didn't notice any pain relief, and put them on a shelf as decoration.

This is not meant to diagnose, downplay, cure, or treat any health condition, disease, condition or illness. However, pure essential oils can support your body systems, relieve symptoms, and enhance your overall wellness strategy when accompanied by other lifestyle changes.

There are times when we feel energetic, alive, full of vitality, at optimum (a high level of) health, and ready to take on the world. Our vibrational frequency is elevated and our body is functioning as it was designed to.

Then there are times when we are "under" the weather, feeling "down" and experiencing illness or dis-ease. Our vibrational frequency has fallen and illness is setting in. Without taking corrective action, we will likely continue to spiral downward and get very, very sick.

115

The metaphorical "dividing line" between the two is the *wellness line*, and what you are learning now will help you live above it.

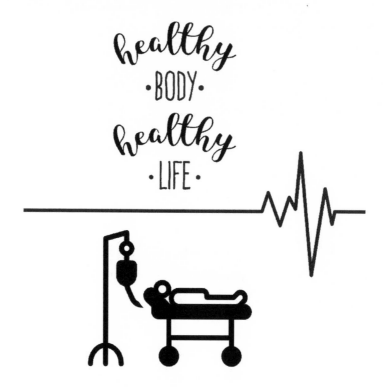

Mindset, diet, exercise, making intentional choices to manage stress and past trauma, and consciously using plant-based products in day-to-day life collectively support the vitality in people you know who are living above the wellness line.

So what prevents you from living this way if it is indeed what you truly desire?

Not having a strong enough conviction to change is one reason. If you aren't sick enough yet, you might put your wellness a little further down the priority list, thinking you have time to get healthy later, or that autoimmune illness won't happen to you. Even after I had two diagnoses that were autoimmune-related, I still didn't take action other than to keep making doctor appointments.

Focusing on all the obstacles rather than how to maneuver around them is another way people sabotage their wellness journey. Self-sabotage is rooted in childhood beliefs instilled in us at an early age. And then often backed up by doctors telling their patients diseases are permanent and have no cure.

Now, I have never said I'm cured from autoimmune disease, but if I'm symptom-free, isn't that the best-case scenario? If lupus and hypothyroid indicators used to be on my bloodwork and now don't show up — but are supposedly incurable — do I still have them? If I was supposed to be on pills for the rest of my life, how am I still alive after four years without taking them? (This is somewhat sarcastic, I know, but then again, I have actually been asked that very question by fellow autoimmune warriors who haven't yet decided to try natural healing.)

Although I have a huge scar on my back from a surgical procedure to remove melanoma, I have known functional medicine doctors to say they have patients living active, healthy, symptom-free lives with some cancers. My original dark mole might or might not have remained the same size once I began my health journey, but I wanted it biopsied. Once cancer is cut into, it's like being opened or "woken up," in a way, and it can begin to spread.

If we can have the quality of life we want, is a cure or cutting out pieces of our body really even something we should be most focused on? So many things are said to not even have a cure at all. So would a better use of our personal and global resources be spent on early prevention and long-term wellness efforts? The time and resources we spend on illness after-the-fact (once we get sick) is mindboggling.

You have likely tried many different ways to improve your health before finding this book, but subconsciously something has stopped you from achieving your goal. Perhaps you don't truly believe whatever you are doing will help in the long run.

Your desire for a better outcome for yourself
must overpower your limiting beliefs
in order for you to succeed.

You can work on changing your narrative and breaking through your limiting beliefs through therapies like daily affirmations, choosing positive language and thoughts, and Aroma Freedom Technique (AFT), which is mindset work with essential oils.

There are quite a few pure-plant essential oils that can help you live above the wellness line, and many support the functions of your endocrine system in general. I used to worry about using immune-supporting oils because people would say certain oils would "boost" my immune system, and yet my immune system was already overactive. Once I realized my immune system was not "high" but was out of whack because my endocrine system was out of whack, it made sense to me to use essential oils to support the wellness I wanted to have.

When you wait until you are below the wellness line, it takes significantly more effort to bring you back up above the line again. I didn't listen to my body's warning signals of complex regional pain syndrome, then hypothyroidism, while also ignoring my chronic stress, eating inflammatory, nutrient-deficient foods, and using toxic products. I was eventually forced to deal with lupus and mixed connective tissue disease, too. And then skin cancer.

How bad does it need to get before you say enough is enough and you deserve a better life?

Everywhere you look, people are willing to help teach about safely using essential oils. I am a bit of a nerd and love reading PubMed articles on essential oils from a science perspective, and I have also taken a 150-hour aromatherapy certification. I truly love to share my knowledge to help others live above the wellness line.

It is a lot to absorb, and frankly I could write an entire book just on how to use oils and which ones I love and why, so I'll keep it as short as possible while still giving you a good idea of how they can help with your wellness strategy.

Key concepts when starting with EOs:

Store-bought (grocery store, big box store, etc.) essential oils (EOs) are generally perfume-grade and not edible (whereas many pure, premium oils can be ingested). Most store-bought oils will also contain instructions not to apply them to your skin. Honestly, with your skin gobbling up everything you slather on it, you should not put anything on it that you wouldn't eat or inhale into your lungs.

Have you gone looking at essential oils and seen that some companies seem really expensive and some are really low cost? Store-bought oils (and the ones sold on Amazon, Wish, etc.) have synthetic fillers to "stretch out" essential oils so retailers can sell them cheaper. The low-cost knockoffs are full of endocrine disruptors and won't do anything for your wellness. In fact, they will *contribute* to your illness.

Source a high-quality brand of essential oils through someone who is knowledgeable about quality, distillation process, farming methods and farming partners that the company uses to grow their plants, and how the oils work. While you'll come across people and online articles putting down social networking and multi-level marketing companies, the truth is their products — oils and everything else — are usually very high quality, and you can't buy them in a retail store because the companies want to make sure there is person-to-person education about the products and usage.

Network / MLM companies usually provide an aspirational amount of training to their members. You'll get as much free education as you could ever want when you get your products through one of their knowledgeable distributors / members / representatives who are working hard to grow their home-based business with integrity and serve their customers in a way no big-box store would be interested in doing. Of course, some reps may be more customer-centered, knowledgeable and helpful than others. You'll know pretty quickly.

If you decide to try a certain essential oil, research credible sources for its therapeutic action and any safety precautions. Essential oils like Rosemary, Wintergreen, Cypress, Clove, Eucalyptus and a few others may lower blood pressure, for example. If you are on medication to lower your blood pressure, and you use an oil known to encourage or support a healthy ("normal") blood pressure level, monitor your blood pressure closely. ("Support" doesn't mean go up — it means it helps get to an optimum outcome.) Talk to your doctor and pharmacist if your pressure drops — the medication and oils may be doubling-up the effect, and you might even be able to choose between pill OR essential oil (with your doctor's approval of course. Never, ever just quit medication without consulting your doctor.) Also be aware a congested liver can cause high blood pressure — optimizing your nutrition with a whole food plant-based diet can also help normalize blood pressure significantly.

Start LOW (1-3 drops at a time) and go SLOW with pure plant extract essential oils — they are undiluted, with no fillers, highly concentrated, and very potent.

High quality essential oils work best when used daily, not used only in times of sickness. Let them help you stay above the wellness line rather than only using them when you're below it.

HOT oils such as Clove, Cinnamon, Nutmeg, or Oregano, and any blends with these oils in them, may need dilution with coconut oil when using on your skin.

Do NOT apply essential oils to your skin immediately after a hot bath or shower as your pores are wide open and some oils will feel uncomfortably hot. Wait at least 30-60 minutes.

Please read the inside labels on your oils and have a knowledgeable mentor who can guide you with safe, proper usage.

Observe your mood when you use any oils and you'll soon discover which ones your body responds to for emotional support, mood enhancement, or even pain relief. It can be challenging to try to convince yourself to use an oil to feel happy, positive, or high-vibing if you really dislike the smell.

Everyone has different preferences, so it's important to try a few different oils when using them for specific reasons.

Constituents are parts of plants that make up the whole plant. Many plant constituents have been studied for their therapeutic actions, or effects on health and the body, so sometimes even though companies are unable to make health claims about what their oils can do because of government regulations, an online search for the constituents in those oils and information on scientific websites like PubMed about specific health benefits will guide you. If you get in the habit of looking up the main constituents of each oil, you'll gain a good understanding of what therapeutic value the oil may provide for your body. Each person is affected in different ways, so be prepared to try a few oils to figure out which ones work best in your body for whatever particular relief you are seeking.

When looking things up on the internet: search for details such as "benefits of Cypress essential oil" or "constituents of Cypress essential oil." (And other oils you are interested in.) If you just type the name of the oil, you'll get lots of ads to buy oils from every supplier on the planet — but what's important when you're first learning about them is to look at what they can "do" which will help you narrow down which ones to try first. Perfumes or synthetic oils won't have any therapeutic action, which is why premium essential oils are so amazing. They aren't for making your house smell fresh — they pack a punch in the health and wellness department!

When you come across articles online, make sure they are referenced and backed up by medical evidence (doctors, pharmacists, pub med research, etc.) Learning for yourself is so empowering. And knowing where to look is important. I did two years of research about essential oils on PubMed, Google Scholar, functional medicine doctor websites, and university websites even before taking my aromatherapy certification. There are over 22,000 articles and studies on the free PubMed website about essential oils, without any brand bias. Anyone can read them, anytime.

Rather than watching TV or scrolling social media, block out some time in your calendar daily to read some science-based articles about various essential oils. There are also lots of free trainings online with experienced aromatherapists.

If you want to be healthier, you're going to
need to do some homework.

NOTES

CHAPTER TWELVE

Liver Health, Inflammation, and Food

Start now; start from where you are.
Baby steps may be tiny, yet they
are forward momentum.

Your liver performs about five hundred vital functions, more than any other organ. It acts as a filter for your blood as well as storing blood and regulating its constituents. The liver's functions range from detoxification to balancing your metabolism.

Some of the liver's jobs are making lipids (cholesterol, triglycerides, lipoproteins) and bile to break down fats. If your cholesterol is out of range, this can be a sign of liver malfunction. Don't just take a pill to manually suppress your cholesterol. High cholesterol is a sign of something else — so a more logical choice is to find the root cause.

The liver stores blood and nutrients (vitamins A, D, B12 and iron), plus dismantles and recycles other substances (old red blood cells and excess hormones). The liver transforms fats, proteins and carbs into usable fuel from foods you eat.

One of the most critical jobs your liver does, however, is removing toxic substances from your blood. Toxins are everywhere, in the air you breathe into your lungs, products you put on your skin, the foods you eat and water you drink. Anything that enters the body ends up in the blood, which eventually ends up in the liver. In fact, the liver filters approximately three pints of blood in a single minute!

Pesticides and other unnatural products (like petroleum-based ingredients) in our food are a large contributor to poor liver health.

As a fellow autoimmune warrior, I know what it's like to feel worn out. I'm sure you are struggling with chronic fatigue, inflammation, and chronic pain. I get it. I was there too, right where you are now. I had days at a time where I had such brain fog I couldn't figure out how to make coffee in the morning, my whole body hurt, I couldn't snap myself out of extreme, limb-weakness exhaustion, and needed a nap within two hours of waking up.

When you're in that state, you go looking for something, anything, that promises to give you a boost. Because wouldn't it be amazing to have an afternoon full of energy so you could feel human again and do all the things you miss doing?

There are companies who prey on chronically tired people. Your tired, struggling self is their target market for their unhealthy product — isn't this awful? Thanks to millions of dollars spent by the companies on their marketing strategies, people think energy drinks enhance energy, improve physical endurance, boost your mood, help you to fly, and speed up your metabolism.

However, serious health risks have been reported with energy drink consumption! Things like heart attacks, strokes, seizures, and heart arrhythmias.

"More than 20,000 emergency department visits related to energy drink consumption were reported in 2011." — American Heart Association

"Energy drinks have been linked to an increase in emergency room visits and deaths." — Journal of the American Heart Association

"The combination of [this specific energy drink] and mental stress impose a cumulative cardiovascular load and reduces cerebral blood flow." — Pub Med: Cardiovascular and cerebrovascular effects in response to [this specific energy drink] consumption combined with mental stress. (Randomized controlled trial)

Marketing is extremely lucrative for companies and they invest millions of dollars to convince you to buy their products. A lot of time, effort and obviously money goes into the subconscious programming companies want to drill into our minds about the dreamy, perfect, energized lifestyle their product can offer us. This goes for all products, by the way. The more picture-perfect their actors' lifestyles look, the more likely consumers are to buy, hoping to feel what the paid actor was brilliantly portraying in the ad.

If you grew up with the "food / dietary guides" telling you protein comes from meat, or if you remember commercials that convinced us milk does a body good, these are hard lessons to unlearn. Contrary to popular belief, protein is not a food group; it's a macronutrient, and is available in a wide variety of plants. Food recommendations of the past have been highly influenced by the meat and dairy industries which are now feeling threatened by the plant-based awakening. Thankfully, Canadian and US governments have both recently published updated guidelines to healthy eating which encourage more foods from plant sources and to limit highly processed foods, saturated fats, trans fats, added sugars, salt and alcohol. The Government of Canada Food Guide website (https://food-guide.canada.ca) also has an entire page devoted to marketing, and that food marketing awareness is a "food skill." Their opening statement says, *"It is important to be aware of marketing because it can influence your food choices."* Education like this is a huge leap in the right direction.

Did you know a single meal consisting of meat, dairy or eggs can trigger inflammation in the body within just a few hours? And that inflammation can even cause cognitive impairment? There are a couple of ways animal products (meat and dairy) cause inflammation: They are high in saturated fat (which can trigger inflammation), and they are a breeding ground for bacterial toxins known as endotoxins, which are inflammatory.

If you study your regular bloodwork results you've probably seen you have been tested for C Reactive Protein, or CRP. CRP indicates the levels of inflammation in the body, and can also help your doctor learn if you are at risk for heart issues. Brain fog is an extremely common issue for autoimmune warriors and inflammation plays a significant role in causing this symptom. In 2013, a systematic review of 46 individual studies found that in meat eaters (Western diet), biomarkers of inflammation (CRP) were frequently higher than normal over those eating a vegetable- and fruit-based diet. *(Pub Med: Dietary pattern analysis and biomarkers of low-grade inflammation, 2013).*

Since inflammation underpins so many diseases, it makes sense that an anti-inflammatory way of eating would be beneficial for our body and our brain. Lowering our inflammation helps us feel more alert, more energetic, with less pain, and fewer symptoms. And yet in mainstream society, plant-based diets (and vegans) are associated with weakness while we are led to believe carnivores are the strong ones. It's so backwards!

If you start paying attention to magazine ads, TV commercials and social-media advertisements, they all grab your attention when you see yourself in their actors and think your life could be that amazing if you only bought their thing. When it comes to the meat industry, they make a summertime BBQ look like the best day ever! There's a happy, smiling dad, flipping burgers or grilling a steak to perfection as all his friends laugh at his jokes. What guy wouldn't see this as the perfect day and want to grab a bunch of steaks, buy a new shiny barbeque, and renovate his backyard?

Effects on the environment aside, the meat industry is contributing to a growing number of health issues, while plant-based alternatives not only exist, but are healthy and taste great. We eat burgers regularly, with patties made from black beans. If you are looking for a meat alternative to help you transition to a plant-based way of eating, "plant-based meats" are a tasty option as well, but be aware they do have added oils in them and some are highly processed.

We need to start getting serious about showing companies how we feel about being duped. You choose where to spend your money — is what you are buying getting you closer to your goal?

If you want to be healthier, use your hard-earned money to purchase products from companies that supply you with pesticide-free, sugar-free, whole foods made from plants.

Food Additives

You've heard about glyphosate for years now, right? It's not only bad for the bees, it's bad for the humans too. Glyphosate — and every other pesticide used in the food supply system — is an endocrine disrupter and destroys the microbiome. If you aren't eating organic food, pesticides and herbicides were used to grow it and are now contributing to your gut permeability (leaky gut).

Then there are food colors. Natural colors used in the food industry come from molecules that have been isolated from plants and insects. However, these are more expensive than artificial colors which come from petroleum. Synthetic dyes can be mass-produced much more cheaply, and were originally made from coal tar. Artificial food dyes these days are now petroleum-derived substances, which still is not a necessary ingredient to be fueling your body with. You wouldn't purposefully add these ingredients to your child's lunch, or to your guests' plates when you invite them for dinner. So why are we so accepting of these things being in "foods" (using the term loosely now) on grocery store shelves?

Research shows consuming Red Dye 40 affects the metabolism of other nutrients and affects brain functioning without crossing the blood-brain barrier. Also, Red Dye 40 contains p-Cresidine, which the U.S.

Department of Health and Human Services says is "reasonably anticipated" to be a human carcinogen.

In the United States, companies are required under the FDA to label dyes used under the list of ingredients. However, Canadian regulations allow for murkiness: Red Dye 40 is called Allura Red on Canadian labels. A pretty name doesn't make it safer.

These colorings are in cereals, drinks (alcoholic and non-alcoholic), dairy products, spices, snack items, baked goods, sauces, as well as in pharmaceuticals and cosmetics.

And other dye numbers have other pretty names in Canada and are equally harmful to our health.

Sugar

There is so much confusion around sugar because the human body runs on glucose, which is a form of sugar. Healthy meals get converted into glucose to fuel our muscles, brain, and entire body.

The problem is the sugar we are most familiar with, granular stuff in a bag, is highly processed. Not only that, but there are numerous varieties of sugar, some with names that even sound vaguely healthy, like "coconut sugar," and "cane sugar." In the vast majority of packaged foods and junk foods, even things like potato chips that you think aren't sweet have all kinds of highly processed sweeteners, often derived from corn but altered so drastically they are unrecognizable to the body and liver.

Processed sugars in all their forms deplete your body of critical electrolytes. Electrolytes are essential minerals in the body that have an electric charge and are necessary for many key functions. They help regulate nerve and muscle function, control the balance of fluids, they play a role in blood pressure, muscle contraction, and if you don't have enough electrolytes, you may feel dehydrated, run-down, or may even experience muscle cramps and spasms.

The irony that some companies sell electrolyte drinks with sugar(s) and colorings is not lost on me. This is yet another important reminder to read labels and understand the ingredients, in order to be able to make better health decisions. This is actually what makes a whole-food, plant-based diet easier: the idea is to purchase lots of fresh and frozen fruits and vegetables, single-ingredient dried foods like beans, lentils, quinoa, and wild rice, and packaged foods with as few ingredients as possible. You can think of it as decluttering your diet.

If you're looking for a natural electrolyte drink, pure coconut water is a great option. If you aren't drinking the water directly from raw coconuts, make sure you are reading labels on drink packages because some coconut water companies do not use organic coconuts and some also add sugar or synthetic sweeteners.

Processed sugars also deplete your body of antioxidants. Antioxidants are molecules that can prevent or slow down the damaging effects of oxidative stress (the imbalance between free radicals and antioxidants). So why do antioxidants matter? Uncontrolled oxidative stress, and excess free radicals, are linked to a number of health conditions including diabetes, hardening of blood vessels, high blood pressure, inflammatory conditions, neurodegenerative diseases, and cancer. Reducing your sugar intake and increasing your antioxidant intake are important not just when battling these illnesses, but to keep your health above the wellness line.

You can increase your antioxidant intake by "eating the rainbow." Focus on brightly colored fruits and vegetables such as blueberries, cranberries, blackberries, wolfberries (goji berries), artichokes, and dark leafy greens, as well as pecans and red kidney beans. I love to blend several of these foods together daily (blueberries, blackberries, strawberries, and kale or spinach) into a nutrient-dense smoothie.

I don't eat a lot of sugar anymore but when I do, I feel hungover for two days afterwards and almost always have significant knee pain. Paying close attention to how we feel (even days later) after the foods we consume can be an important motivator to reduce our intake of obvious foods that cause excess inflammation or other uncomfortable symptoms.

Sugar can also cause spikes and drops in blood glucose level, and interfere with immune function, causing you to get sick more often and more severely. If you feel a cold coming on, cut out all sugar immediately.

Sugar feeds bacteria and parasites, like yeast and Candida. It also depletes your body of good gut bacteria, promoting leaky gut and other gut infections. Chronic pain, vision problems, and even wrinkles can be worsened by sugar. While cancer can move in when the immune system is malfunctioning, sugar causes cancer cells to reproduce and thrive, and blocks mechanisms that would slow down or kill cancer cells and tumors.

Sugar (in all its many forms) is an addictive ingredient very few people are worried about. And yet you can see it's a significant health threat. Do you know what to look for on labels? This not an all-inclusive list but ingredients to avoid are:

- White sugar
- Granulated sugar
- Brown sugar
- Cane sugar
- Corn syrup, corn sugar, corn sweetener
- High fructose corn syrup
- Coconut sugar
- Invert sugar
- Syrup sugar molecules ending in "ose" — dextrose, sucralose, fructose, sucrose, glucose, lactose)
- Fruit juice concentrates

Don't be fooled into thinking the zero-calorie sweeteners are a better choice. When aspartame is broken down by the body, some of it produces methanol, which degrades into formaldehyde, a carcinogen and neurotoxin.

A quick online search in Google Scholar shows numerous science-based articles about health concerns from using aspartame. This ingredient is used in thousands of foods as well as pharmaceuticals, and has been linked to headaches, strokes, heart issues, neurotransmitter imbalance, cognitive abnormalities, systemic inflammation and epilepsy.

If you want a sweetener, use honey, maple syrup or date paste, but don't overdo these either. There is no physiological need for our food to be sweet — our body creates the glucose it needs.

Gluten

Gluten is a group of seed-storage proteins found in many grains, but the majority of gluten sensitivities come from eating wheat. The first time I went "wheat-free," it was for three months and it wasn't easy. I was shocked at how many packaged products contain wheat in some form or fashion.

Gluten in wheat gives dough its glue-like elasticity, helping it rise and hold its fluffed-up shape. If you've tried gluten-free bread, many brands have had a hard time imitating the feel and texture we are used to; it's common for gluten-free bread products to have a denser, heavier texture.

A growing number of people have realized gluten causes them to have inflammatory and autoimmune reactions. Symptoms of gluten sensitivity range from irritable bowel symptoms, chronic fatigue, headaches, fibromyalgia symptoms, eczema, and rashes, to neurological disorder symptoms like muscle weakness, poor coordination, loss of sensation, confusion, brain fog, and pain.

When you read that list of symptoms aren't they eerily similar to many autoimmune conditions? Could the answer be as simple as cutting out gluten to prevent some or all of these symptoms?

Simple, and yet not easy. Have you ever heard someone say going gluten-free is a fad, or that people are doing it just to be trendy? If you have ever tried to go completely gluten-free, you'll immediately realize no one does this for fun. It's extremely difficult to avoid gluten, and people who are gluten-free are often shamed by their friends and family for "being difficult" at family gatherings and then are guilted into eating foods with gluten in them just to be polite.

Action steps you can start today:

Get clear on why you want to be healthy. Write your reasons down in a journal or on a sticky-note where you can see them. What would it mean for your enjoyment of life if you didn't have symptoms anymore?

Get out your calendar. Commit to a minimum of 30 days, ideally 60 days, to eliminate toxins and improve your diet. Be specific: Commit to going gluten-free, or eating organic, or cutting out all forms of sugar for a period of time. See how you feel after 30-60 days and adjust your diet and lifestyle from there.

Set yourself up for success by planning ahead. If you know you give up easily because you are overworked and too busy, make a meal plan you can manage with your schedule. There are lots of websites and social media foodies that share all kinds of great, printable recipes. With technology and research literally at our fingertips, there is no reason you can't do this if you really want to.

What do you want your life to be like in 60 days? The same? Frustrated and battling all your symptoms, having had read this book but still contemplating what to do and not doing anything? Procrastination is self-sabotage, by the way. So is continuing to eat foods that you know cause uncomfortable or painful symptoms. If this is all too familiar to you, now is a great time for more mindset work and journaling to explore what limiting beliefs may be holding you back and why.

Does it seem like an unrealistic idea? Could changing what you eat help at all?

The great news is it's free to try. All you need to buy is grocery store food and you already buy that anyway. In fact, it's cheaper to eat whole foods from plants, and make your own meals. In the grand scheme of things, 60 days is not an unreasonable amount of time to do something for your health that could open up a new future for you. One without inflammation, pain, chronic fatigue, frustration and despair.

NOTES

CHAPTER THIRTEEN

Plant-Based Nutrition for the Win

Your future depends on what you do today.
You either make yourself miserable or
you make yourself strong. The
amount of work is the same.

D o you want natural, sustained energy? Of course you do. Anyone with a chronic illness or busy household wants that desperately, sometimes above all else. Here's the thing though: It isn't a one-time drink in a can. It isn't hiding in a secret supplement or vitamin.

There is no quick fix and even when you feel better, you still need to continue with the lifestyle in order to stay above the wellness line.

This is exactly why "diets" don't work — because people think when they reach the end goal they can go back to their old, unhealthy habits without consequence. There's always a consequence.

Hopefully you realize now that inflammation goes hand in hand with many chronic diseases. I used to wonder if the disease came first and caused the inflammation, or if the inflammation (from something else) eventually caused the disease. By the time I had four autoimmune conditions I was at my wit's end and just wanted to feel better again. I desperately wanted my life back.

If your goal is wellness and to get better from symptoms you are struggling with, buying unhealthy, inflammatory, low-quality food wrapped in several layers of plastic is a form of self-sabotage, not to mention a complete waste of money. I have practiced intentional spending for the last fifteen or so years in other areas of my life, but I didn't make a connection to my grocery bill until the last couple of years. Let's start spending our hard-earned money on stuff that is good for us, helps us be better versions of ourselves, is more economical, and helps live above the wellness line.

Buying healthy food makes more sense because you get more bang for your buck — you are fueling your body, you'll feel noticeable improvements within a short timeframe, and you'll be improving your long-term health.

Plant-based nutrition is what our
bodies require for optimum wellness.

It was the meat and dairy industry that convinced us animal products were required in our diets. Whole-plant foods are loaded with phytonutrients that offer anti-inflammatory effects. They help your body heal naturally from the inside out, while simultaneously putting a lid on inflammation.

The compounded effect of ditching inflammatory
animal products AND eating an anti-inflammatory,
whole-food, plant-based diet has helped people
naturally eliminate many symptoms related
to diabetes, rheumatoid arthritis, lupus,

cognitive disorders, thyroid imbalance,
psoriasis, and many other conditions.

Additionally, increased fiber intake (like from chickpeas, lentils, and other beans/legumes) helps improve bowel health, helps lower cholesterol, helps control blood sugar levels, helps lower your risk of heart disease, and more.

Now, do I believe you can heal from autoimmune illness just with diet change, while still using toxins, sabotaging yourself with unprocessed emotions, and practicing a negative mindset? No.

You can improve your gut health and therefore your overall health to a certain degree by eating a whole-food, plant-based diet. But your vibrational energy and emotional health are just as important for your complete wellbeing. And if you continue using synthetic products in, on, and around your body, toxins will continue to accumulate inside you.

So, back to your diet: The best way to avoid unwanted additives is to eat real food. Not packaged, processed stuff. Look for everything to have as few ingredients as possible, and don't believe what's on the front packaging. I once bought sugar-free ketchup thinking I was doing myself a favor. When I got home and looked at the ingredients, it had artificial sweetener in it: a synthetic product even worse for our health than real sugar.

Breakfasts are more healthy (and filling) if they are real oatmeal (cooked steel cut or rolled oats), or cooked quinoa with organic fruit. If you need it to be a little sweet, add a spoonful or two of real maple syrup (not corn syrup). Many pre-packaged, flavored "instant" oatmeal cereals are loaded with sugar, salt, and a thickening agent called calcium stearate (which, according to a National Organic Standards Board Technical Advisory Panel Review, can cause abdominal pain, dizziness, and ringing in the ears, among other alarming symptoms). Another great reason to stick to plain, organic steel cut or rolled oats and add your own fruit.

Another great breakfast idea is quinoa homemade bagels (oil-free, gluten-free, and compliant with a whole-food, plant-based way of eating). Add some natural, organic, pure peanut butter (just peanuts) and slices of organic banana, and even your kids will want some!

These are significantly more biologically appropriate fuel sources than boxed, dried, sugary "crunch" cereals with bits of "fruit flavored" puffs that are colored with health-concerning dyes and loaded with a paragraph of ingredients you can't pronounce.

On a whole-food, plant-based, no-oil diet, even "sweets" can be made healthy. Dates (the fruit) are great all by themselves! Or homemade applesauce (if you buy applesauce rather than making it yourself, check it doesn't have added color, sugar, or anything else.) Mike and I both love our sweets, so I love making goodies like sweet potato brownies, peanut butter cookies, or vegan chocolate lava cakes, for example. If we don't feel like making dessert, dates dipped in peanut butter are a favorite go-to.

It's possible to still satisfy your sweet tooth without compromising your health. You'll also find you have fewer cravings once you start fueling your body properly.

If you want to start and aren't sure how, do some vegetarian meals between your regular ones. And when you do eat meat, eat only half your usual portion, and add extra sides of plant-based dishes (beans, legumes, vegetables, and fruit). Aim to eat 10-15 servings every day of fruits and vegetables, and fill rest of your diet with complex carbs like potatoes, sweet potatoes, gluten-free pasta, legumes, wild rice and beans. Eating this way will leave you very little room for meat and will be a much easier transition than just eating cold salad for every meal.

As I already touched on, the "fake" meats on grocery store shelves these days are a helpful option during your transition, but just like Oreo cookies, they are in the category of vegan junk food. I love using this example because, clearly, Oreos are not healthy. But they are vegan! Fake meats are highly processed and full of oil. They are not considered "compliant" with a true whole-food, plant-based (WFPB) no-oil diet, but they can be a helpful crutch to help you get over any frustration of what to make for dinner, and to get your spouse and kids on board with switching to eating more plant-based meals.

Start reading labels, and start eating more whole foods — real foods. It's important. And when you search online for vegan recipes, just omit any added oils as well. Oils will eventually clog up your blood-flow pathways.

Our bodies actually require very little fat, and we have been duped into thinking it is good for us, and that we can free-pour it on our salads, in our frying pans, in our baking, and dip our breadsticks in it. I get all the healthy fats I need from whole foods like nuts, olives, coconuts, peanut butter, and avocados, and I eat a wide variety of foods every day, at every meal, that are filling and help improve my health naturally.

If you believe you can't do it, you'll be right. I hear this often. People tell me, "Sure, you do it, but I can't eat that way." (This is self-sabotage, in case you missed it.) My response is, "Why not?"

More often than not, their answer is buried in excuses.

- *No time to look up and plan a new recipe.*
- *No desire to spend 30 minutes prepping dinner before cooking it.*
- *No emotional energy to expend on doing anything new.*

This comes down to mindset, pure and simple.

We set our priorities based on what matters to us most. Change might feel uncomfortable. But so does staying where you are, doesn't it?

If you were happy with your health, you wouldn't be looking for help. You are deserving of feeling healthier. I know you're reading this right now because you desire a change — and because I've done it, I know you can too.

Can you imagine what daily life would feel like if you didn't have pain or even minor annoyances from inflammation?

There are a great number of people with chronically clogged sinuses, or who suffer with frequent headaches, and when they remove all dairy (milk, cream, butter, sour cream, cheese, and yogurt) from their diet, these symptoms clear up, sometimes within just a week or two. Other people have found eliminating gluten is the secret to preventing migraines. No matter what symptoms you have, your body is telling you it isn't happy. If you get any symptoms regularly, or even on occasion, isn't a diet change worth trying? Even if you feel like you can't give up these things, there are lots of healthier plant-based, and gluten-free alternatives.

Action steps — the trifecta summary:

The key to sustained energy, which will give you back a sense of normalcy in your day-to-day life, is achieved by:

- learning more about and cultivating proper gut health with a balanced, whole-food, plant-based, no-oil diet;
- proper daily hydration with good quality, pure water;
- detoxification of your entire lifestyle (your products, your food, and your emotions); and
- taking steps to heal from past trauma and intentionally managing your chronic and daily stress.

Do you see the entire trifecta represented here?
Mindset, products, and nutrition.

If I were to sum up my entire recovery
into one concise list, this is it.
This is what I did, and
I know you can do it, too.

Aromatherapy

Specific to feeling more energetic naturally, if you would also appreciate a "wake up" essential oil, Rosemary, Eucalyptus Globulus, Peppermint, Black Pepper, Lemon, and Lemongrass can be very useful, each on their own or in combinations.

You can't outrun the negative consequences of a bad diet with just adding in some essential oils, but Mike and I both find these ones helpful if we need a little "pick-me-up." We make nasal inhalers with eight drops each of Rosemary and Black Pepper essential oil. It's a healthy way to combat the odd afternoon slump, with zero calories, and we know lots of shift workers who say this combination helps them fight off drowsiness on night shifts.

Blank nasal inhalers can be purchased online for about a dollar each. 15-16 drops of essential oil may cost another couple of dollars. So for less than five dollars per inhaler, we get at least three or four months of use out of each one.

NOTES

CHAPTER FOURTEEN

Wellness Takes Guts

Eat like you love yourself.
Nourish yourself with goodness.

The gut, which includes the small and large intestine, is the largest immune organ in mammals. As an infant, you got your gut flora at birth from your mother. Whatever state her microbiome was in, that's what you started out with. From then on, it's heavily influenced by the lifestyle and eating habits of your parents. In adulthood, your microbiome is a result of your own choices which, let's face it, are heavily influenced by your engrained habits from childhood.

The study of our microbiome is relatively new in the realm of scientific discovery. And what doctors and scientists are learning is mind blowing. Our gut flora is a collective healing agent capable of doing battle with autoimmune diseases like multiple sclerosis, lupus, rheumatoid arthritis, diabetes, and more.

Gut health and liver health keep our heart functioning properly. Remember I mentioned high blood pressure can indicate a congested liver? Now that you know this, do you think popping a blood pressure "suppression" pill will fix it? A pill manually forces blood pressure down, but it's like using a piece of duct tape to hide a festering wound. It doesn't address the root problem. A 3-day fast to reset your liver is a much better option, as recommended by many liver experts — it's a quick, cost-effective and pill-free way to see what that does for your blood pressure.

Digestive enzymes in the gut are molecules activated by stomach acid. They help break down protein into small peptides and amino acids, break down fat into fatty acids, and break down carbs into simple sugars. Commonly used over-the-counter and prescribed medications that are wreaking havoc are antacids and proton-pump inhibitors (PPIs) used for indigestion, heartburn and acid reflux. They reduce the amount of acid in the stomach and yet we *require* acid to digest food and keep the microbiome balanced.

In the words of Dr. Daniel Nuzum, who has a Ph.D. in Naturopathic Medicine and Mechanotherapy, and a second Ph.D. in Natural Medicine, *"The best way to ensure that you will develop an autoimmune disease is to reduce the acidity of your stomach."*

Gastric acid helps keep harmful bacteria at bay so, not surprisingly, when people take antacids or PPIs, their food is not being properly digested, the bad bacteria begin to flourish, and additional health issues arise.

When gut health is compromised, the thin membrane lining the gut becomes more permeable; partially digested food particles along with toxins and bad bacteria end up being absorbed through the intestinal walls and entering the bloodstream. The body thinks these particles are foreign invaders and attacks them, causing inflammation, joint pain, fatigue, malabsorption of nutrients (including Vitamin B12 and magnesium), acid reflux, heartburn, food sensitivities, and other autoimmune symptoms. Many autoimmune warriors experience these symptoms; there is a direct link between gut health and autoimmune illness.

Toxin accumulation due to poor air quality inside and outside (chemical pollutants), lower oxygen levels (spending more time indoors in winter), Franken-food (highly processed and genetically modified), high-sugar snacks, treats and drinks, and pharmaceuticals, all force the liver (the body's filter) to work overtime.

Speaking of poor-quality nutrition, did you know there is a nutrient link to thyroid hormone production? Every cell in your body relies on the thyroid hormones for metabolism — converting oxygen and calories to energy. Without adequate iodine, zinc, and selenium from foods in your diet, your thyroid can't convert T4 to T3, and as you know, T3 is the gas in your tank. You don't just feel sluggish in a way that can be ignored. You are running on fumes and it's not sustainable for much longer.

All these things have choices attached. What we put in our mouth — in the form of food and pills — has enormous consequences. We can be intentional about our health or we can be lazy about it. We can choose to be outside more or we can choose not to. If you suffer from heartburn, indigestion or acid reflux, these are symptoms that many people find disappear on their own with a better diet — one that is whole-food, plant-based, oil-free. This means you wouldn't need the bandaid approach of the antacids or PPIs. Halting a natural bodily function (your digestive acid) has consequences that can be dire. Preventing symptoms from happening at all leads to an improved quality of life for those I know who have done it.

We can choose to eat more organic foods, eat whole foods, and avoid nutrient-lacking junk foods, or we can sabotage our health for whatever reason. We can purify our indoor air with a diffuser, use only natural cleaners, and change our furnace filters — or not.

Ladies, in menopause our ovaries will begin to fail, if they haven't failed already. Because of their failure, we will no longer produce at least five hormones including progesterone, testosterone, estradiol, DHEA, and pregnenolone. These hormones not only make us beautiful women inside and out but keep our emotions balanced and protect us from the symptoms of aging.

What does this have to do with gut health? You can help balance your hormones naturally through improving your gut health, which can be quite helpful in lessening the challenging symptoms of PMS in our early years and menopause in our later years.

Migraines, heartburn, PMS, hot flashes, poor sleep, acid reflux, and all kinds of other regular everyday things that people have come to think of as normal are actually red flags. These symptoms mean your "check engine light" is on. Your body is struggling. Healing your autoimmune and endocrine systems requires healing your gut as a main priority.

Make time for your wellness before you are
forced to make time for your illness.

We really have a huge amount of control over our health, it's just that sometimes we wait for a life-interrupting malfunction before we pay attention.

Sleep

It may feel like we're getting off track here but I promise you, there's a strong connection between gut health and sleep.

Sleep is a time to restore and regenerate.
It's your body's time to heal itself,
physically and mentally.

While it used to be thought that you could "catch up" on sleep on days off after a busy work week or busy month with little or irregular amounts of sleep, experts have realized the concept of sleep debt (and trying to repay that debt on the weekends) isn't an appropriate way to look at this area of your health. It's like eating junk food all week and then saying you've caught up on your health by eating salads on the weekend.

Let's be honest. Your body can't stay above the wellness line if this is your strategy.

We are diurnal creatures and have a circadian rhythm that has evolved over millions of years. Our hunter-gatherer genetic heritage means we are designed to wake up with the bright sun, be physically active (outdoors) in the warmer daytime, and sleep when it gets dark and cooler. Our circadian rhythm affects our body's core temperature, hormone production, brain activity, cell regeneration, and other important biological processes.

In today's era, we spend the majority of time indoors under artificial lighting, in recirculated or stuffy air, and keep our thermostats set at the same degree 24 hours a day. Even "daylight" bulbs will never be actual sunshine. This type of environment doesn't let our body know the natural circadian rhythmic cues it needs for optimized function.

A healthy adult should be sleeping somewhere between seven to nine hours each (and every) night, and wake up feeling refreshed. When you're fighting autoimmune illness, there is a lot going on beneath the surface: inflammation, brain fog, pain, taking pain killers throughout the day, feeling emotionally numb and hopeless, reaching for "comfort foods" to try to feel some sort of brief pleasure rather than making healthier choices, taking antacids for the heartburn, and then needing a couple of glasses of wine or sleep medications just to get some rest. I know, because I've been there.

While autoimmune warriors are often feeling completely exhausted, it's extremely common to not get quality sleep. When is the last time you slept through the night (without sleep aids), and woke up feeling refreshed, excited, and ready to take on the day?

A good night's sleep doesn't happen automatically, as you probably know all too well. And keep in mind I'm talking about real, natural sleep, not sedation from pills or alcohol.

There needs to be a strategy during the daytime, with nighttime in mind. A consistent bed time and wake time are fully within your control if you pre-plan and make sleep a priority.

So how does this relate to food and gut health?

Getting your digestive system regulated and cleaned up can greatly improve your overall health including sleep quality. Since sleep is regenerative, it can then lead to an improvement in your overall health, mood, pain levels, energy, and can even improve your skin health.

Between 10 p.m. and 3 a.m. your body repairs, restores, and regenerates hormone balance, skin health and texture, your gallbladder (specifically between 11 p.m. and 1 a.m.), and your liver (specifically between 1 a.m. and 3 a.m.). If you wake up regularly during those windows of time, your body may be trying to send you a message that it needs help in that particular area.

There is no shortage of things we can look at that will help optimize our sleep, gut health being one of them. And since poor gut health, poor liver health, and poor sleep go hand-in-hand with autoimmune illness, hopefully you can see why this is a key area to focus on to kick-start your healing.

What can you do to help with sleep and gut health together? A lot!

While most of us can't change the fact that most of our daily lives are spent indoors, try to mimic nature by making indoor lighting and temperature adjustments to correlate with bright light, fresh air and warmer temperatures in the daytime, and dim lighting and cooler temperatures at night.

Don't eat after dark. Eating after dark would not likely have occurred in our earlier evolutionary days because we would go to sleep when the sun went down.

Properly hydrate in the daytime (do not wait till bedtime to drink a bunch of water). I drink a bare minimum of 1 liter of water daily (approximately a quarter gallon), sipped throughout the day, and I aim to drink 2 liters daily (approximately a half gallon) as my ideal goal. Your hydration requirement will also depend on the temperature, how active you are, how dry your environment is, your diet, if you are pregnant or breastfeeding, your current state of health, and what medications you may be taking.

If you drink or eat anything with caffeine, limit your caffeine intake to mornings. If you drink caffeinated beverages in the morning to fight off feelings of grogginess, try going outside into sunlight instead, so your body's natural nighttime melatonin production gets halted (as it is designed to naturally do in sunlight).

Avoid endocrine-disrupting pesticides and preservatives in your food/drinks which can cause hormone imbalances that interfere with your sleep cycle (eat whole foods, limit the packaged and lab-made stuff).

Cut back on or eliminate all the processed sugars.

Eliminate fatty meals (they are really congesting for your liver, gallbladder, arteries and heart).

Eat well: whole foods, plant based. This way of eating isn't boring, so don't worry about that. We still eat our favorite meals like pizza, shepherd's pie, pasta, chili, fajitas, burgers, and more, all without inflammatory meat or dairy. When we make a stir fry, we fry the vegetables in broth rather than oil. Even things like mayo, "cheese" sauces and salad dressings can be made completely from whole-food, plant-based ingredients, and without dairy or oil.

Eat natural sources of digestive enzymes: mangos, bananas, papaya, avocados and honey.

Make sure you're taking a high quality multi-B vitamin daily.

Exercise (with the approval of your doctor) can improve mental clarity during the daytime, helps burn off the problematic stress chemicals, and can greatly assist with quality sleep. A stretching and strengthening program such as yoga can also help improve your flexibility, reduce tension, and can release tight muscles. Please erase the saying "no pain, no gain" from your vocabulary. If you have not been regularly exercising, make sure to start slowly and if you feel pain, back off. Pain is one of your body's warning signals that something is wrong, and it is important to pay attention to.

Speaking of physical movement, chiropractic care is a self-care tool that can help with restful, deep sleep and overall health and comfort. In addition to spine inflammation, misalignment can cause pressure on nerve roots and cause pain in the immediate area, or the pain can radiate elsewhere. Pain is hard enough to cope with sometimes during the day, but adds insult to injury when it prevents you from sleeping. Spine and joint adjustments can be helpful to reduce pain, and improve mobility, circulation, blood flow, nerve health and immune function.

The nerves coming from the vertebrae connect the brain with the rest of the body, and can affect various body parts and systems. This became evident to me when I had digestive issues on a day I also happened to have a chiropractor treatment booked. I was feeling bloated and "backed up," like things just weren't moving through my system. The chiropractor felt my spine alignment to determine where to adjust me, and on this particular day my mid-back was having some new issues. He asked me if I had been having any stomach or digestive problems and I was surprised, and a little embarrassed. *How could he tell I was constipated by touching my back?* Well, apparently my vertebra that was out of alignment was pressing on nerves connecting to my stomach and digestive tract. Possibly for days. After my adjustment, the flow-through noticeably improved!

A happy digestive system helps you sleep better, and one of the most important (and often forgotten) organs is your liver. With a close link between poor liver health and autoimmune illness, as an autoimmune warrior, it would be very wise for you to move "liver health" to the top of your list of priorities.

Vitamin C is a potent antioxidant, an excellent liver support supplement, and can be used as a cleanser to help the liver repair itself naturally. Since there is very close correlation between poor liver health and autoimmune conditions, I use the powdered form (sodium ascorbate, without any added calcium) to be able to take large quantities of it daily.

Intermittent fasting is also very beneficial for the liver. The easiest period for most people to fast (me included) is between dinner the night before and lunch the following day.

Probiotics (and probiotic foods) help the digestive tract return to a balanced state, and the stomach will naturally be able to produce the acid it needs. Probiotics are living strains of bacteria that add to the good bacteria in your gut. The dairy industry would love for you to believe you can only find probiotics in yogurt but this is not the truth. Since dairy is inflammatory, and contributes to a variety of health issues, it's important to look to other sources for your probiotics. You can buy probiotics in pill form, but an even better place to get your probiotics is by eating an organic, whole-food, plant-based diet. Probiotics are found in fermented foods like sauerkraut, tempeh (we use this in place of bacon in BLT sandwiches), kimchi, kombucha, miso (there are lots of great meal recipes, soups, and even desserts that use miso), and pickled vegetables.

Prebiotics are also necessary (to activate and feed the good bacteria). Prebiotics are in organic bananas, broccoli, apple cider vinegar (many people find taking a small amount of ACV before a meal helpful for digestion and preventing indigestion), onions, garlic, honey, berries, chick peas, lentils, red kidney beans, oats, peas, asparagus, almonds, pistachios, and flaxseeds.

Antibiotics are bacteria killers. You know this. But they kill even the good ones in our gut and digestive tract. Everything. Your entire microbiome gets completely wiped out whenever you take antibiotics. Every single time. This leaves you wide open and very susceptible to a whole host of health issues for months afterwards, which can turn into chronic illness and a vicious circle of always "getting sick" because your microbiome is severely compromised.

If you catch a cough, cold or flu, do you really need antibiotics at all? I've been to doctors who asked me if I wanted them, and I've said yes, thinking it would be helpful. But they really weren't. Antibiotics don't work for viruses and all they do is wipe out your healthy gut flora. This is profoundly counterproductive to good health. In all my trips to multiple doctors for antibiotics over the course of my lifetime, I was never informed of what was really going on inside my gut when I took antibiotics or used an antibacterial ointment on my skin for an infection, or to try to calm a deep itch sensation I randomly experienced (many autoimmune warriors also complain of itchy skin that seems to not be helped with medications). Most people don't realize the influence of the gut over day-to-day quality of life until they heal it and their health issues clear up — and only then it becomes glaringly obvious.

So what can you do instead? Many essential oils have anti-microbial, anti-bacterial, and anti-fungal properties, but what's even better is to prevent illness in the first place.

Living above the wellness line means being free from bladder infections, coughs, colds, athlete's foot, pain, inflammation, ear infections, sinus infections, allergies, bronchitis, skin issues, fatigue, digestive malfunctions, and everything else you can think of that isn't optimum health.

Remember that retina hole I mentioned? I recently learned it sealed a perfect little ring of scar tissue around itself. The eye doctor said a new hole usually means emergency surgery to create scar tissue with a laser, but instead my body healed itself sometime over the last few years. Now, could my body have done that anyway? Perhaps. But if I had continued with my prior unhealthy lifestyle, I don't believe my body would have been able to heal anything on its own. But within six months after my accident I was off medications and eating a more vegetarian / flexitarian diet. For the last two years I have included wolfberries (goji berries) in my diet which have been studied for their positive effects on eye function, and in 2019 I went fully whole food, plant based.

I've avoided antibiotics now for several years, when I used to be on them almost monthly. I was also a queen of disinfectant surface sprays and wipes, strongly scented laundry detergents, dryer sheets, scented beads for my washing machine, vanilla fragranced candles (candles are a double-whammy to your indoor air quality and your endocrine system because of the "fragrance" and smoke), bleach, and plug-in air fresheners (now there's an oxymoron — they are not freshening, they are adding toxins to your air). Looking at this list, it was completely normal for me to use all of these things every day, or every few days, for many years. My body was screaming for a break, and I wasn't listening until autoimmune disease finally had to hit me like a freight train.

Please listen to what your body is trying to tell you. Are you experiencing mild symptoms and feel like you are still somewhat healthy? Imagine being told five years from now that you have lupus, and knowing that there's a good chance you could have avoided it by focusing on preventative and therapeutic health measures? Are you quite sick now, possibly already with a named diagnosis? Imagine being told five years from now that your chronic disease doesn't show up on your bloodwork anymore. Let my trip to hell and back with my four autoimmune diagnoses, and my research into natural ways to heal be your guide to living your life above the wellness line.

Self-sabotage ends here!

Be intentional. Next time you have a meal, drink, or grab your go-to snack, ask yourself if it's something your liver and microbiome will function better with. Will it help or hinder your sleep quality? "You are what you eat" isn't just a meaningless cliché. Your physical health is a direct result of your choices, and you choose every day what to put in your mouth.

Set yourself up for success. If you appreciate reminders, put a note on your fridge door, and at the top of every grocery list. If you will be eating out, plan your meal ahead of time so you make a healthier choice than whatever you used to order.

Mitigate risk. If you or your loved ones absolutely must take antibiotics — if there is no other choice — then rebuilding the microbiome quickly with high quality probiotics is imperative. Otherwise, it's like removing the antivirus software on your computer and opening an internet browser with zero protection.

Aromatherapy

Premium essential oils I use for:

My digestive support (for the rare times I get heartburn, indigestion, upset stomach, diarrhea, bloating, or discomfort): Peppermint, Ginger, Tarragon, Fennel.

My liver support (the body's digestive filter): Grapefruit, Geranium, Helichrysum.

PMS and to prepare my body for a healthy, symptom-free menopause transition: Frankincense, Cedarwood, Bergamot, Peppermint, Wild yam root extract, Clove, Spruce, Pine, Lavender, Clary Sage, and Myrtle (these can be helpful on their own or in combination blends).

Helping me get a better night's sleep: Lavender and Cedarwood together, or Black Spruce.

NOTES

CHAPTER FIFTEEN

Choose the life you live. Don't settle for it.

D o you remember a character in Sesame Street named Guy Smiley who hosted *Here is your life?* When I was little, I didn't know that this was a spoof of a reality documentary for radio and TV called *This is your life,* but I always enjoyed watching the Muppet characters re-live the people, events and experiences that had made them who they were. The segment of the show was meant to teach kids how things were made, but all I knew was that it was inspiring. At some point, I decided that I wanted to be satisfied and proud when I got old if Guy Smiley were to come along and have me sit down for my own episode of *Here is your life.*

By my teen years, I was striving for an adventurous life. One of my earliest crazy adventures was that I was offered an opportunity (and gladly accepted it) to be in a circus act when I was about twelve years old, standing on the muscular back of a beautiful, big white horse as it cantered around the ring in front of a small-town crowd. I was safely secured with a harness attached to pulleys and ropes, and it was exhilarating.

I definitely have experienced ups and downs in my life and got myself into loads of trouble by allowing the wrong people into my circle. I navigated a complicated path of domestic violence in more than one relationship. I made poor choices thinking I was doing something exciting. I overused alcohol, lost friends because of my behavior, and got myself into personal danger at times. My summers of allowing myself to get sunburned increased my risk of melanoma significantly. We all learn from our mistakes and I take responsibility for every single one of my choices: the good, the bad and the ugly.

> *However, I intentionally choose to not dwell on the*
> *poor choices I made. I have learned from them, and*
> *go forward knowing I can choose to do better.*

What didn't change is that I love doing something brave, out of the box, and unexpected. Not because I want the fame or recognition, but because it reminds me to be excited about being alive.

Don't get me wrong, I'm a lover of routines and list-making. I'm also a homebody. An introvert, too. I appreciate lots of alone-time to reflect and recharge.

And yet, I've been cage-diving with great white sharks. It had been one of my only bucket-list dreams, long before I ever heard the term bucket list. My dad took me to the drive-in to see *Jaws* when I was ten years old, and I loved it. I asked for books about sharks for my birthday. I always wanted to see one up close and in its natural habitat. For someone who needs the security of knowing how things will work out and is fearful of traveling solo, I even surprised myself when I got on a plane alone and flew to San Diego. I took a taxi to the marina, got on a live-aboard boat with a group of strangers, headed out to sea two hundred miles off the coast to Guadalupe Island, Mexico, and for the next five days I jumped into a cage in the water multiple times a day with what most of society has been led to believe are man-eating, savage killers.

That trip gave me enormous confidence that I really was capable of doing anything I set my mind to. This is an important lesson to remind yourself of every once in a while.

Then there was the year Mike and I decided we should move to Nicaragua and build a vacation house on a remote Caribbean island. How crazy does that sound? We sold our tiny condo on Vancouver Island, BC, bought a cargo trailer to tow our household stuff in, and only told a handful of people before we left. Our adventures on our drive from Canada to Nicaragua were plenty. We had challenges and laughs as well as just enough danger to make for some entertaining stories in the years since!

Before we left Canada, I renewed my prescriptions as a "just in case" measure. I had started weaning myself off most of them in the months leading up to our trip but wanted to have them if needed. I didn't know how hard it would be to find a doctor and get these medications, but when we arrived in Nicaragua's capital city, I had a full-blown bladder infection and I needed something I hadn't brought with me.

I didn't know yet that antibiotics were so detrimental to gut health, and even if I had, the pain from the infection had me worried. I had already tried to just flush it out with extra water for the previous few days as we drove our way through El Salvador and Honduras, but my bladder discomfort was increasing by the hour. Having had a kidney infection in prior years when I wanted to try to avoid antibiotics, I was not interested in taking that risk again. We learned quickly that you can walk into a pharmacy in Nicaragua and simply ask for what you need. No doctor visit needed for antibiotics!

I say "simply ask" but I don't speak Spanish yet, so I had to type the explanation of my problem into a translator app on my smart phone and show it to the pharmacist. The pharmacist (typing her reply into the app) offered me three different antibiotics, and they were so cheap I bought them all. My doctor in Canada had advised me over the years that it's best to alternate antibiotics and not use the same one over and over. I figured I would need more in a couple of months anyway because I got UTIs so frequently, so I figured why not stock up while I could? We were about to spend the next many months on a small island where supplies were limited.

The antibiotic I decided on for the first treatment was a one-dose powder that I added into some juice. It didn't taste like anything, and I felt better within hours. I felt totally fine by the next day. We've been led to believe Western medicine is the be-all and end-all for "health" care, but this was where I really began to wonder about the bigger picture. Honestly, I was a little bit resentful that this quick fix wasn't available to me until this point. I had suffered with chronic, frequent, painful bladder infections for years. Many other autoimmune warriors suffer from them too. To find relief within hours and with just one dose was mind boggling to me, so I was very grateful.

This was late 2016, and was the point in time my body really began to heal. With all of the lifestyle changes I have made, I am very pleased to say that I haven't had a bladder infection since. If you suffer from frequent infections, hopefully this gives you some additional motivation to create your own lifestyle changes.

While on Big Corn Island, we didn't set alarm clocks. We woke up at sunrise and went to bed within about an hour of when it got dark. Within a few weeks of our arrival, Mike hired a small crew of guys to work with him to clear our two acres of land and 1,500 feet of road through the jungle, all by hand (swinging machetes). This is a remote island in Central America with limited machinery, and every job is labor intensive. To build our house, concrete was mixed in a pile on the ground, by guys with shovels, and using buckets of water coming from a neighbor's hose. It was all very primitive and "back to basics." There was no machinery other than some power tools we had brought with us.

An islander friend of ours came over one day because he knew we had a certain type of wild plant (Cerasee) growing on our land. He asked if he could take some to send on the little puddle-jumper plane to his diabetic mother on the mainland, because she couldn't get it there. He said it "helps clean the blood." We of course told him he could have as much of it as he wanted — to us it was just a weed that we would chop down anyway. We were still in the frame of mind that things for health came in a package or a pill that you bought at a store or pharmacy.

We ate fresh, tree-ripened fruit with every meal. Passion fruit, known on the island as "ca-la-la" gave me a noticeable energy boost for the day when I ate one or two in the mornings. We drank a lot of smoothies for breakfast (and sometimes lunch), with whatever fruits were ready for picking like starfruit, papaya, pineapple, sugar mangos, mango rosas, hairy mangos, big mangos, regular bananas, red bananas, and monkey bananas. I bet you didn't know there is more than one type of mango or banana! We drank lots coconut water and tamarind juice — I later discovered tamarind is known to be a helpful liver detoxifier, so along with our cleaner diet, I was cleansing my liver without even realizing it.

Lunches often consisted of ripe veggies in a huge salad, and dinner at our rental house was usually a pasta dish or fried plantains, because it was quick and we were exhausted from being at the job site all day. This was definitely not a vacation. We had given ourselves some tight timelines to get our house built, and there was no resting.

If we were too tired to cook and went out to eat, it was a treat to eat Italian pizza baked in a wood-fired brick oven (which didn't give me a stomach ache like pizza in Canada), or we would have local Caribbean fish or lobster with rice.

Within the first two months of being in Nicaragua, I was able to finally wean off the last, lowest doses of all my medications completely. These included gabapentin for nerve pain, hydroxychloroquine for lupus, levothyroxine for hypothyroidism, bupropion for depression, mirtazapine for sleep, and over-the-counter naproxen for the day-to-day aches and pains. In past years I had also used prednisone (a corticosteroid) and rounds and rounds of antibiotics for so many infections.

I was finally free. My side effects were fewer, my energy was improving, I wanted to rest in bed less and less, and I no longer needed afternoon naps. I was pretty sure my liver and kidneys were doing a happy dance.

After years of frequent nausea every other day, it completely disappeared. I walked to and from our property building site multiple times a day, I drove around the island shopping in the hardware stores for materials the guys needed, we had a newly rescued, very sick puppy I was taking care of, and I was on the go all day long. The weather was hot and humid, and the sweat poured out of us from sunup to sundown. To cool off before bed, we either went for a swim in the salty Caribbean sea, or showered in cold water (no one has hot water tanks!), and either way we didn't complain.

Before our trip, my friend Megan Bailey gave us a DIY all-natural essential oil bug spray. I quickly realized that it worked really well. Since I was wearing shorts and flip-flops every day, I needed to be able to put it on my skin, and I also sprayed it on our dog, so I was thankful it didn't have chemicals. As it turns out, one of the main ingredients, lemongrass oil, has numerous health benefits: it can help relieve pain, aid in digestion, and is known for its calming, yet energy-boosting effects.

We got used to eating two or three servings of dinner every night. We were so physically busy all day long, every day of the week, that we were starting to wonder how to keep the weight on. My stamina was back to normal, like before I got sick. I felt great!

My body was finally back in a regular sleep cycle, too — sleeping when it was dark and being awake when it was light. This is how humans were designed. My years being awake most of the night were over and done with. I slept like a log, every single night. I woke up refreshed and energized, ready to take on the day. Even now, four years later, I still sleep this well. By the time we returned to Canada, Mike had lost 40 lbs., and I was down 18 lbs.

Sure, you might be thinking I'm suggesting you move to Nicaragua. Don't worry, I'm not. You can do a lot of these things anywhere.

It's within your control; it's up to you.

Spend as much time outside as you can. If you work from home, set up a desk or workspace in an outdoor area if possible, or beside a window that opens, so that in nice weather, you are getting lots of sunlight and fresh air in the daytime as you work. If you have kids, get them outside too! It's the best thing for them — it burns off excess energy, gets them inhaling fresh air, and is good for the whole family's health, physically and mentally, to spend time out in nature together.

Go for walks — several each day, out in the country if at all possible. Or at least near some trees or a body of water. The rhythm of walking, hearing your footsteps on the ground and deep-breathing in nature is amazing as a meditative activity and stress reliever. If you aren't well enough to go for a walk, just go sit outside and breathe in the fresh outside air for half an hour a couple of times a day.

Exercise to get the blood pumping and to work up a sweat. Whether you can manage walking, running, biking, lifting weights, or if you're more into gentle yoga or even chair yoga, DO some form of movement for strength and cardio, every day. Sweating also really helps to detox your body and skin. While I arrived in Nicaragua having not been very active, my body gradually adapted — and after seven or eight months, I was in great shape, wasn't tired at all during the day, and fell asleep as soon as my head hit the pillow at night after my cold shower to cool off from the sweaty temperatures. Sleep is a game-changer for healing. As are exercise, fresh air, and eating real, whole foods.

Speaking of sweating to detoxify, and knowing that sea water has healing benefits, here's a great salty ocean recipe for an evening bath: equal parts (1/2 cup each) of baking soda, salt (sea or Himalayan pink), and Magnesium Epsom salt (make sure it's the organic, non-fragranced type). Have a 40-minute soak several times a week and make sure you hydrate during and after by drinking extra water.

Eating well will lower your toxin load while adding proper nutrition — a win-win. My diet in Nicaragua changed based on local, available fresh foods. When I began to feel markedly better, I took stock of exactly what we were eating: very little beef or pork because it was hard to find on the island, and therefore expensive compared to other foods. We sometimes ate chicken or fish, and had fresh-caught lobster occasionally, but mostly lots of veggies, fruits, rice and beans. The bread we bought at local stores for sandwiches was made with coconut flour, not wheat, and didn't give me any more stomach aches! Wheat is highly inflammatory and most of the world's wheat now (other than Einkorn) is hybridized with significantly more gluten in it. We ate tree-ripened coconuts, passion fruit, bananas and mangos every day (full of helpful digestive enzymes).

Detox through elimination of household toxins. We did our laundry by hand and hung our clothes to dry. We didn't use any dryer sheets (we didn't have a washing machine or dryer.) The sun and wind dried our clothes. Ditch your household chemical cleaners (including bleach) and switch to white vinegar, lemon juice, essential oils, and 100% plant-mineral cleaning and laundry products. We use vinegar and baking soda regularly, and we also buy a 100% plant-mineral household cleaner once or twice a year from the company we get our hand sanitizer and essential oils from. The cleaner is toxin-free, with no endocrine disruptors, it cleans thoroughly, and it is very cost-effective.

If you want some additional resources to be able to dive deeper, I created a detailed autoimmune course, and it's available on my website through the URL address at the back of this book. The course is complete with audio files and videos, links to scientific research to back up everything I have talked about in this book, with greater detail provided in the course, as well as functional medicine and plant-based websites, social media accounts to follow for tasty, compliant meal recipes, DIY natural cleaning recipes, and more. It's all you'll need to turn your health around if you feel you need more specific direction and guidance.

With autoimmune illness, everyone is at a different stage of health function or malfunction. At one end of the spectrum, you might not realize you are heading for illness. You might not feel it yet. You might be hovering just above the wellness line, and the littlest thing could knock you down.

As you continue your toxic lifestyle and eating habits, piling on the daily stressors and trying to swallow your constant emotional triggers, you dip below the line.

You might have headaches, skin issues that seem to have no explanation, occasional bouts of dizziness, or an odd day of feeling really run-down, but have been fighting through it and pushing yourself onward without making any lifestyle adjustments.

Every symptom is a result of suboptimal function and shouldn't be ignored; it's your body's way of trying to communicate with you.

As you inch further down below the line, you will start to really struggle. As your health continues deteriorating, you may wake up one morning and not be able to go to work anymore, or hold down your dinner, and you are scared that your body might really be shutting down this time.

Your body may be malfunctioning
but it's not defective. You are not broken.

You have developed new self-management skills
and you think differently now.

Go forward, knowing you have the capacity,
discipline and resilience to recover quickly
from difficulties in your life, with
self-awareness and purpose.

I believe everything happens for a reason, whether we can see it in the moment or sometimes not until years later. You picked up this book for a reason. You read through each and every page, knowing this is exactly what you needed right now.

You learned about the trifecta — the *perfect storm*. You deepened your self-awareness and emotional intelligence by determining your core values, your superpower, ways to build your resiliency, what your motivations are and what matters to you most, along with the outcomes and consequences of taking action vs. doing nothing.

You expanded your knowledge, you trusted the process, and it brought you here.

You thought you were going to discover your x-factor and instead, you discovered nine of them that fit together in your personal matrix like pieces to the most complex puzzle you've ever put together.

You have a well-stocked toolbox now — all the tools you need, and your very own master key.

It's time for you to unlock it.

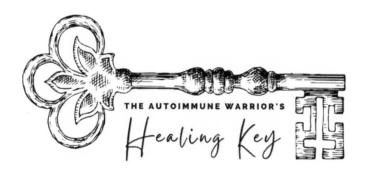

NOTES

ABOUT THE AUTHOR

Jo Pronger Faulkner is an animal lover, nature enthusiast, avid reader, photographer, drama and negativity avoider, sprinkler of sarcasm, straight talker, and Caribbean dreamer. Jo encourages women to listen to their intuition, step into their personal power and design the life they want, with oomph and gumption.

Her favorite quote is, *"Whether you believe you can do a thing or not, you are right."* (Henry Ford)

Jo lives in Northwestern Ontario, Canada, with her fiancé Mike, and their hilariously opinionated dog Jemison.

BONUS RESOURCES

Looking for the link to the printable files mentioned in this book?

Type this URL address into your web browser:

https://JoProngerFaulkner.com/taiwhkbr2021

You will also find links on that webpage to Jo's in-depth autoimmune course, where to find her on social media, join her private groups where she shares positive mindset tips, stress-management techniques, whole-food, plant-based recipes, autoimmune education, essential oil tips, and other helpful resources and products.